CHICAGO PUBLIC LIBRARY

R02018 86613

BUSINESS/SCIENCE/TECHNOLOGY DIVISION
CHICAGO PUBLIC LIBRARY
400 SOUTH STATE STREET
CHICAGO, IL 60605

# Scleroderma
## THE PROVEN THERAPY THAT CAN SAVE YOUR LIFE

*HENRY SCAMMELL*

*M. EVANS AND COMPANY, INC.*
*NEW YORK*

Copyright © 1998, 2003 by Henry Scammell

All rights reserved. No part of this book my be reproduced or transmitted in any form or by any means without the written consent of the publisher.

M. Evans and Company, Inc.
216 East 49th Street
New York, New York 10017

LCCN number: 97-061593

**Library of Congress Cataloging-in-Publication Data**

Scammell, Henry
    Scleroderma : the proven therapy that can save your life / Henry Scammell.
    192 p. ; 23 cm
    Includes index
    ISBN number: 1-59077-023-4
    1. Systemic scleroderma--Chemotherapy. 2. Systemic scleroderma--Etiology. 3. Antiboitics. I. Title.
    [RC924.5.S34S27 1998]
    616.5'544--dc21

DESIGN AND TYPESETTING BY RIK LAIN SCHELL

Manufactured in the United States of America

9  8  7  6  5  4  3  2  1

## ASK YOUR DOCTOR

This book does not substitute for the medical advice and supervision of your personal physician. No medical therapy should be undertaken except under the direction of a physician.

If it has been medically determined that you are suffering from scleroderma, your physician should have the opportunity to read this book, to learn about the infectious etiology of the disease and its treatment with the safe, clinically tested and proven therapy that it describes.

# CONTENTS

# The Need to Know

This book describes the disease that almost killed me, and the therapy that really did save my life. At the time I started treatment, I doubt if one scleroderma patient in ten was aware they even had a choice. In fact, at some stage in our stories, that is one of the main things that everyone with this illness has in common: not knowing.

In my case, that not knowing began in mid-1986, the day after my fortieth birthday, with the first signs that something was going wrong in my body. There were changes in my hands . . . pain in my fingers . . . swollen joints . . . the first subtle stiffening of the skin. I had done a tour in Vietnam as a Marine, but that was 18 years earlier; it didn't seem likely there was any connection to what was happening now. My doctor was concerned, and when he couldn't put a name to it he sent me to a rheumatologist. The specialist diagnosed me with mixed connective tissue disease and prescribed some of the standard drugs then in use for rheumatoid arthritis. But whatever it was kept getting worse. After a couple more referrals over the next two years, I was finally diagnosed with systemic scleroderma. It's a rare disease, but this last doctor recognized it the minute I walked into his office. He told me not to worry about it, but by amazing coincidence I saw a television show that same night in which I learned the systemic form is the most often fatal.

The usual pattern for scleroderma is that the symptoms peak at around the end of the second year after onset, and then stabilize at a slightly lower level of activity for the rest of its course. I reached that plateau at around the time of my diagnosis, and although the scleroderma didn't seem to be getting any worse, nothing the doctors gave me made it any better. In fact, over the following decade I suspected my body was suffering as much damage from the medications as from the disease. One of the drugs was prednisone, which the doctors initially prescribed at 80 mg a day. Despite the medicines, the scleroderma entered my esophagus. In 1995, in large measure because the drugs had disarmed my immune system, I developed tuberculosis. I had trouble swallowing, the prednisone had turned my skin to paper, and I was reduced to a 105-pound skeleton who needed help just to stand. It was the closest I came to dying.

In early 1998, a scleroderma patient named Pat Ganger came to Cincinati to talk with a local support group about her disease. She told us that the International Society for Rheumatic Therapies was going to hold its annual meeting in Boston in another few weeks, and that the results of a small but important study would be presented at that meeting. Pat was a founder of The Road Back Foundation, which had sponsored the study at a teaching hospital of Harvard Medical School. She gave me an advance copy of two new books, both by a medical writer named Henry Scammell. *The New Arthritis Breakthrough* described the use of minocycline in connective tissue diseases in general. The other book was this one.

I started poring over *Scleroderma* in the car as my wife drove me back from that meeting, and when we got home I didn't stop reading until I was finished. If Pat Ganger was an example of what to expect from the treatment, I could hardly wait to get started. Pat had given me the telephone number of Dr. David Trentham, the physician who had overseen the study. I called him the first thing the next morning, and he agreed to see me right away at his office in Boston. A few days later he presented his paper at the medical meeting, and CNN broadcast the story of this therapy around the world. By then I already had my first small clues that I was on the road to recovery.

Now, almost 5 years later, although there is still scar tissue in my esophagus, I can swallow with ease, my skin is healthy again, my weight has come up to normal, my muscle tone has returned, and I'm back to fulltime work. Perhaps the biggest miracle of all is that I have been able to return to an important pastime that I had thought was gone forever—the game of golf. The therapy has not only restored my health, it has returned the quality of my life.

I'm also grateful that this experience has included the chance for me to give something in return. I have made a pledge to do all that I can to spread the word to everyone with the need to know, to promote more research, and to ensure that others are able to gain access to this treatment that has worked so well for so many.

If you or someone you love suffers from this disease in any of its forms, I hope this book will be a first step,

as it was for me and many others, on the road back to
a full and healthy life.

—Russ Elliot, President,
The Road Back Foundation

## PROLOGUE

This book is about the search for the cause and cure of a fatal disease, and about how we are connected in the chain of life.

Scleroderma, a connective tissue disorder which means "hard skin," is rare, probably afflicting fewer than half a million Americans. Because it can be extremely cruel, and since there is new evidence that it may be spreading rapidly, it has become one of the most compelling enigmas in medicine.

Just how compelling was demonstrated at a recent annual scientific meeting of the American College of Rheumatology (ACR). Some two thousand physicians, or about half of all the doctors attending that year's meeting, filled the aisles and overflowed into the halls outside one of the largest of the auditoriums for a presentation by leading researchers in scleroderma.

The way things then stood, the doctors were told, a diagnosis of that disease was equivalent to straddling the bannister at the top of a long stairway. No matter what was done to intervene—regardless of the skill of the physician or the choices from the small arsenal of medicines used to treat it—the forces of nature would pull the patient irresistibly down the railing, which gradually but inevitably turned into a razor blade.

Whether it was too lurid or because it was not entirely original, that depressing metaphor never found its way into the ACR's summary of the presentation. But none challenged its relevance to a hopeless prognosis.

That evening another presentation, on new modalities in the treatment of rheumatic disease, offered a telling contrast to the downbeat outlook of scleroderma. The focus was on the MIRA study (for minocycline in rheumatoid arthritis), the subject of a tantalizing preview to the general assembly on the opening day. It would be hard to imagine a subject more central to the stated purposes of the ACR.

The session, like several other study groups, was assigned to a small, hot, claustrophobic room in the cellar of the conference center. Not only was it held at night, but the timing conflicted with the free annual gala hosted by one of the major pharmaceutical firms. As the band played far above, only a relative few physicians and researchers at the conference eschewed the airy vastness of the ballroom to answer a call to duty down among the steampipes. Those who attended the seminar on new modalities—fewer than two hundred and most notably from the United States, Israel, and the Netherlands—spent an intense two hours comparing their successes with a safe, simple, inexpensive therapy that had proven in clinical trials to be dramatically effective against rheumatoid arthritis.

The answer to scleroderma was also in that room. Like so much else that passed there, lacking the powerful advocacy and financial support available to medical therapies that produce great profit, it would remain unheard and unexamined by all but a few.

Its time would come.

# CHAPTER ONE
# First Light

Shortly after noontime on Tuesday, the sixth of August, 1996, two physician-researchers presented the preliminary report on an open-label study of minocycline therapy on eleven patients with early diffuse scleroderma to the study's sponsors at a small French restaurant in Brookline, Massachusetts. Veronique's is on the ground floor of an older, mock-Gothic apartment complex called Longwood Towers, just across Brookline Avenue, the MBTA trolley tracks, and the Fens from Beth Israel, the principle teaching hospital of Harvard Medical School. The audience for the report was three trustees of The Road Back Foundation. There was room to spare at the circular table.

Some of the group had been looking forward to this moment for years. Because the study's sponsors were from out of town, they had initially rendezvoused with the two doctors in the Beth Israel lobby. No specific early results from the study were discussed in the short trip through the Fens, a bucolic link in the famous Green Necklace around the city of Boston designed in the mid-nineteenth century by pioneering landscape architect Frederick Law Olmsted. But expectations were high, and during that walk the jovial tension continued to accumulate between the researchers who held the secret and the visitors who would soon share it.

The hopes of the Foundation members for this study were based mostly on their own experiences and the kind of untested case histories physicians call "anecdotal evidence." Pat Ganger, the Foundation's director, had herself been diagnosed with scleroderma thirteen years earlier, and her case was one such seminal story.

For the first several years of her disease, Pat had been treated with conventional therapies from an armamentarium of powerful agents developed initially to fight cancer or malaria. During that period, her symptoms had steadily worsened. Rather than suffer the side effects of drugs that were producing no apparent benefit for her illness, she quit them all and founded a support group of scleroderma patients in the Columbus, Ohio, area to share the meager data available on their disease and to support each other while facing an outcome that appeared inevitable.

A year later, a member of that group told Pat about a book she had just read by Thomas McPherson Brown, M.D., director of The Arthritis Institute at Washington's National Hospital. *The Road Back* described a different therapy for a number of rheumatic diseases, based on safe, simple antibiotics in the tetracycline family. Pat went to Washington, and in short order Dr. Brown's protocol put her scleroderma into remission.

Diane Aronson, whose life had been interrupted almost thirty years before by severely crippling rheumatoid arthritis, traveled to this day's meeting along a similar path to Pat's. After hearing about Dr.

Brown's therapy and *The Road Back* in 1987 on a segment of ABC's *20/20*, she had gone to Washington and started treatment at the National Hospital. Her symptoms began to slowly improve, and over the following years the frequency and severity of her arthritic flares diminished steadily, although not with the dramatic finality of Pat Ganger's scleroderma.

In the late 1980s, Diane and a lady she had met in Washington named Jane Fagan were among the first of Dr. Brown's Boston arthritis patients to transfer their treatment to Beth Israel Hospital. Their new doctor, who was familiar with Dr. Brown's work and was willing to follow a similar protocol in providing the same therapy, was a rheumatologist named David Trentham.

Every disease that has ever been cured through the scientific study of an observed clinical effect involves stories similar to Pat's and Diane's. But not every physician is as willing as Dr. Trentham to listen to the patient. Instead of seeking out such experiences and systematically examining them for the insights they might provide to the healing process, paradoxically the institution of medical research treats anecdotal evidence as so suspect and unreliable that the term itself has become anathema. No matter how numerous, consistent, or compelling the stories, physicians who offer even the most benign therapies based on such untested clinical evidence may be subject to bans and penalties by the full ecclesiastical court of their peers, including a painful, crippling, sometimes fatal form of professional excommunication.

All his credentials and accomplishments notwithstanding, Dr. Thomas McPherson Brown had endured such a fate, in a classic Catch-22 that began when the government withheld research funds and then the medical establishment attacked his credibility because he was unable to conduct and analyze the kind of clinical tests that would support his case. His therapy was vindicated at last by the minocycline in rheumatoid arthritis (MIRA) trials. A multimillion dollar study funded by the National Institutes of Health at six research centers throughout the United States, including Harvard Medical School, its results were reported in *Annals of Internal Medicine* in January, 1995. But by the time publication of the study began restoring Dr. Brown's reputation, he had been dead for almost seven years.

His co-author of *The Road Back*, however, was still alive, and as a trustee of the Foundation, I was the third member of the visiting trio of sponsors. My hopes for the scleroderma study, like Pat's and Diane's, were twofold: it would validate the anecdotal evidence, some of which had been included in our book, and prove minocycline can cure this usually fatal disease; and, in so doing, the study would provide another model for the efficacy of antibiotic therapy for connective tissue diseases in general.

In the eight years since beginning our collaboration on *The Road Back*, and particularly since Tom's death, I had encountered hundreds of patients. Among them, they represented just about every one of the ailments covered by the book. Some contacted me because they were looking for a local doctor who could provide the therapy, while others who had already taken it wanted to thank someone for their improvement. Those latter calls were obviously meant for Tom Brown, and I accepted them as his proxy. A high number of them came from people who had recovered from scleroderma—far fewer than from arthritis, but more in proportion to the relative rarity of the disease.

Tom Brown wouldn't have been surprised. He knew from his clinical experience that minocycline was effective in relieving or remitting rheumatoid arthritis in some 75 to 90 percent of the patients who persisted in the therapy, but the process could take months or even years. By contrast, he estimated that he had treated some forty patients suffering from scleroderma, which is far less common, and to his best knowledge *all* of them had improved or remitted, some dramatically reversing their disease process in a matter of only weeks. He was quick to point out that he had never done a follow-up study, and patients who have to travel long distances are not always faithful in reporting a good result when their initial motive in contacting a doctor has been removed—or in reporting a bad result when therapy fails. While he considered diffuse scleroderma to be inevitably fatal unless the patient dies of something else first, he never lost a single patient to the disease who completed the antibiotic therapy under his supervision.

Shortly after *The Road Back* was printed, Dick Kislik, a vice president with M. Evans and Company, the publisher, called to report that a doctor from Boston had given a paper in Arizona in which he discussed rheumatoid arthritis as an infectious disease. That had been the prevailing view of rheumatoid arthritis up through the 1940s, but in parallel with the rise of cortical steroids and other anti-inflammatories starting after World War II, it became obvious the process was more complicated. Steroids worked so well on the symptoms of rheumatoid arthritis, at least until they created symptoms of their own such as cataracts and kidney failure, that it was assumed (incorrectly) that the drugs were addressing the cause of the disease. So the baby got thrown out with the bathwater, and by 1988 the infectious theory had come to be regarded by most physicians as an anachronism or a joke. Kislik knew it was the central premise to Tom Brown's use of antibiotics, and he passed along the doctor's name in the thought I might learn something from him that could boost the book.

That's how I came to meet David Trentham.

By then the infectious theory had become hugely politicized, and it was tempting in those days to believe that every rheumatologist besides Tom Brown was an enemy to the concept of antibiotic therapy, so I approached our initial contact gingerly. When I finally tracked Dr. Trentham down at Beth Israel Hospital, where he was head of the department of rheumatology and an associate professor at Harvard Medical School, any such apprehensions disappeared in a moment. He was welcoming and friendly, and although he pointed out that an infectious etiology for rheumatoid arthritis was still a long way from being proven, it was clear he was not among the researchers still snickering at the concept. In the following months, Dr. Trentham met in Boston with Dr. Millicent Coker-Vann, research director of the Arthritis Institute, and he subsequently flew to Arlington, Virginia for a tour of the Institute's laboratories at the National Hospital.

In early 1990, less than a year after Tom Brown's death, Dr. Trentham sent me a paper from *The Journal of Rheumatology*, written by a Dutch physician named Ferdinand Breedveld, reporting on work he had begun while he was one of Dr. Trentham's research associates at Beth Israel. "Minocycline Treatment for Rheumatoid Arthritis: An Open Dose-Finding Study" discussed his experience with ten patients in the Netherlands who had taken oral minocycline for sixteen weeks.

*Half of the efficacy variables improved significantly after four weeks of therapy. At the end of the study, all variables were significantly changed compared with their pretreatment values. We conclude that minocycline may be beneficial in RA. This effect needs to be confirmed in controlled studies.*

Dr. Breedveld's research had a lot going against it: it had been conducted outside the United States on a small patient base without placebos or double-blind controls over a time span that some researchers would dismiss as trivially short. Its publication in a leading American medical journal inspired instant controversy, and the resulting attention proved to be an irresistible wedge in opening the door that had been welded shut for so many years against Tom Brown and antibiotic therapy. Some years later, Dr. Breedveld's study would provide the model for a similar research project, this time on scleroderma, proposed and funded by The Road Back Foundation with contributions from around the world.

Ours would be conducted in America, and the time frame would be a more credible forty-eight weeks. Because scleroderma is a fatal disease, we had ethical misgivings about the use of placebo controls on a treatment we knew could bring remission, so the proposal requested by The Road Back Foundation was for an open study, which meant every patient in it would receive the same medicine, administered to the same protocol. We agreed to a similar number of patients to the group studied by Dr. Breedveld.

Because of its size and timing, Dr. Trentham told us he would be assigning the study to a young Australian rheumatologist who was soon to arrive for a one-year fellowship as a research associate in his department at Harvard Medical School. We knew that in addition to Dr. Trentham's large clinical practice, plus a steadily growing number of assignments from the National Institutes of Health and contracts with private industry, he was committed to even more responsibilities as president-elect of the recently formed International Society for Rheumatic Therapies. A research fellow, working under his close supervision, seemed an ideal solution.

Some fifteen months later, with the study nearing completion, Dr. Trentham introduced us to Dr. Christine Le in the lobby of Beth Israel. We'd had very little tangible feedback up to that point beyond hearing that the study was going very well, and as our group of five crossed Brookline Avenue and walked down into the Fens on our way to lunch, all three of the sponsors examined Dr. Le in much the same way we might have studied leaves in the bottom of our teacups for clues to what lay just ahead—and with much the same result. Both she and Trentham were animated, clearly enthusiastic, polite, attentive, encouraging, even openly optimistic. But it wasn't until we were finished with our club sandwiches that Dr. Le quietly reached down into the briefcase beside her chair and distributed five copies of a short document entitled, "Minocycline in Scleroderma: Open-label Study of Eleven Patients with Early Diffuse Scleroderma."

She invited our attention to the page headed *Patient Profile*. "As you know, the study was designed for ten patients," she began, "and this report shows eleven. One of our original subjects had cancer at the time of her enrollment, and even though her scleroderma improved significantly with the minocycline, it soon became apparent she would not survive the cancer for the term of the study. When an opportunity presented itself, we added an eleventh subject in January; four months later, the cancer patient died."

We all looked down at the profile, searching for the two patients in question. Line five was a seventy-four-year-old female from Massachusetts who had been referred to the study by a rheumatologist. The table listed her skin score at the time she entered the study as 32, fairly high out of a possible maximum of 51. (The modified Rodnan total skin thickness score in systemic scleroderma is the sum total of clinical measurements at seventeen sites on the body, rated on a scale of 0 to 3 for normal, mild, moderate, or severe thickening.) By the time of her first follow-up the score had dropped by nearly half to 17, and three months later it was down to 10. But that was the last visit her cancer would allow her to make, and the line ended with the notation that she had died on May 2. The eleventh patient was a fifty-four-year-old male from Texas.

Dr. Trentham pointed out that those changes were more than a matter of subtraction and addition. The cancer patient could not be taken out of the study just because she had died of another cause than scleroderma, and the eleventh patient could not be viewed, from a statistical viewpoint, as her replacement. It also meant that the date of the final enrollment would correspondingly extend the study's closing date to somewhere around the end of the year.

Dr. Le took us through the rest of the profile. Two of the remaining patients, one with an initial skin score of 43 and the other with a 33, had such severe scleroderma that they experienced kidney failure and had to seek dialysis almost at the start, well before the first follow-up visit, a protocol violation which made it impossible to assess their response to the minocycline and precluded their continued participation in the study. Another patient, a fifty-three-year-old woman from Maine, violated protocol when she took an additional therapy for an oral yeast infection (a relatively minor effect sometimes associated with the use of antibiotics); her entering skin score was 20, at the first follow-up it was down to 4, and at the second visit, just before she treated the yeast problem, it was within a single point of remission. But the violation took her out of the study from that point on, and "almost" doesn't count.

The only other drop-out was a thirty-one-year-old male from Pennsylvania who entered the study with a skin score of 33 and went up to 35 by his first follow-up. The young man had come to Beth Israel on a referral from The Road Back Foundation, and Pat Ganger knew the case personally. He was still on antibiotics but had left the study because of a switch in the route of administration from oral to intravenous (IV) therapy in the hope of saving his life.

Six patients of the original eleven were expected to complete the study. Of the two who already had, one had started at a skin score of 43 and after downward fluctuations by as much as 17 points had finished at 40, for a final result of virtually no net improvement. The second, a forty-two-year-old female from Connecticut, started with a skin score of 33, descended to 22 at her first follow-up, 20 at her second, and 4 at the third; her skin score at the time of the final visit was zero, and she was in remission.

Two of the four remaining subjects had similarly attained remission before their final visits. One, a thirty-two-year-old woman from Maine, had gone from a starting score of 15 to 7 at the first follow-up and zero at the second. The other was a fifty-seven-year-old woman from California who started with a score of 25, had two visits at 5, and reached remission by the third.

The skin scores of the third patient, a sixty-five-year-old woman from Canada, went from 20 to 15 to 13 to 10, with her final visit scheduled for just a week from the date of our meeting.

The last patient in the study was the Texan, who had started that January with a score of 15. He had dropped to 6 in his first follow-up, then to 2, and with two visits still to go was expected to end up in remission as well.

So, of the six patients who had finished the study or were about to, five had improved substantially, with a probable four of them achieving full remission.

The first Netherlands study had helped start a revolution with far less dramatic evidence that minocycline therapy is a safe, effective treatment for rheumatoid arthritis. In all the long history of scleroderma, there had never before been any other therapy that even came close to achieving these results.

## CHAPTER TWO

# Portrait of a Disease

Nobody knows how long scleroderma has been around, but the first medical description of the disease is believed to have been written two-and-a-half centuries ago in southern Italy by a Dr. Carlo Curzio. In the summer of 1752, a young woman of seventeen was admitted to the Royal Hospital in Naples, where Curzio was a physician. Her appearance was frightening, the skin of her face a mask so tight and leathery that it had lost all ability to form an expression, the mouth a ragged, shrunken, immobile hole that exposed her teeth. The same condition prevailed over most of her body; the skin of her neck was bound as rigidly as a drum, and she could barely nod or turn her head.

Over the following eleven months, Dr. Curzio treated his patient with warm milk, vapor baths, and small doses of quicksilver (mercury), the latter two therapies also being among the standard treatments at the time for syphilis. His description of the case, written in 1753, includes a happy ending for the original symptoms with restoration of the natural suppleness and softness of her skin. But it can be assumed that by then the young woman's body had absorbed enough quicksilver to severely damage most of her internal organs and unwrap the wiring of her central nervous system, so we can only speculate on how fully she appreciated her deliverance or indeed how long she lived beyond this "cure."

The disease didn't get its name until almost a century later, when Elie Gintrac of Bordeaux, France, classified it as a skin disease.

Today scleroderma remains a frightening and mysterious affliction, with only the most speculative understanding of its cause, how it is transmitted, or even its frequency. It presents in a number of ways, most of them involving anomalies of the skin, and the various forms are generally divided into two categories: systemic, or diffuse; and the less serious limited versions. Because it would be too expensive to find out how many people have it, not even the United States government's Center for Disease Control in Atlanta, Georgia, keeps any numbers. Estimates by others run from as few as 100,000 to as many as a million. Most researchers believe the number is somewhere short of the middle, between 350,000 and 500,000. Four times as many women get the disease as men, and proportionally more blacks than whites contract the most deadly form. The majority of its victims are between thirty and fifty years old.

Scleroderma is apparently becoming more prevalent, but there is no consensus on how fast. A retrospective study published in 1997 showed that the incidence of diagnoses in Allegheny County, Pennsylvania between 1973 and 1982 was double the frequency for the previous decade. This could mean any number of things: that diagnostic techniques in the second decade were twice as reliable as in the first; that medical record-keeping was that much better; or that victims had become more willing or able to seek treatment. It could also mean that scleroderma has an environmental component and there is something in the air or water or food of Allegheny County and other places with similar patient clusters that either transmits the disease or triggers a predisposition—and is getting worse. So the doubling may be just a fluke, or it may mean that scleroderma is becoming one of the fastest-growing diseases in America.

Because scleroderma presents as a skin disease, for many years it was handled principally by dermatologists. In recent decades, however, with improved appreciation that the systemic form predictably involves a number of internal organs and probably the immune process—analogous to rheumatoid arthritis or lupus—the primary responder has become more likely to be a rheumatologist. Most dermatologists weren't sorry to see it go; scleroderma is considered to be untreatable by either specialty, and nobody likes to work with patients they can't help.

Only rarely does scleroderma afflict families, and although a handful of such cases have been reported in the literature, they are few enough to be explained by shared environment or even random chance. In the case of identical twins in which only one had scleroderma, pronounced differences in lymphocyte function also minimize the probable role of genetics in the predisposition to the disease.

The evidence for a possible environmental connection, however, may be somewhat more substantial. Exposure to silica dust multiplies the risk of the disease, with a study in (then) East Germany reporting that males with silicosis, or black lung, were 110 times more likely to also come down with scleroderma.

Other environmental contaminants associated with the disease include vinyl chloride, organic solvents, biogenic amines, adulterated rapeseed oil, L-tryptophan, silicone breast implants, and the drugs bleomycin and pentazocine.

Whatever its cause, scleroderma has a slow but inexorable evolutionary nature which often culminates in death. The actual percentage of patients who survive long-term remains uncertain, but the most widely cited recent study of patients with diffuse, or systemic, scleroderma, which is the most serious form, shows that nearly two-thirds die of it within ten years.

In its early stages, scleroderma can be difficult to diagnose, not only because it's rare and therefore improbable, but also because many times the early manifestations mimic other, more common diseases such as rheumatoid arthritis or lupus.

Most of the time, a patient developing scleroderma begins to have spasms in the small blood vessels in the ends of the extremities, especially the fingertips and toes, when exposed to cold. This is called Raynaud's syndrome, and although in most cases it does not lead to scleroderma, it can be a harbinger for other symptoms of the disease which begin to surface within the coming months or year. Nine out of ten scleroderma patients experience this phenomenon, with the skin turning waxy-white, or changing rapidly from red to blue.

Less frequent, but also related to blood flow in the affected skin, is a condition called telangiectasia, caused by the dilation of smaller blood vessels which show as small, red or brownish spots on the extremities and face, even inside the mouth.

Probably the most common next symptom is diffuse arthralgia, or aching in the joints, most noticeably in those located furthest from the trunk of the body: the fingers, feet, ankles, wrists, and elbows tend to become painful and stiff, especially early in the morning. This aspect of the disease accounts for the frequent misdiagnosis—or provisional diagnosis—of the disease as rheumatoid arthritis. As a rule, this error is corrected when other manifestations surface which link those early symptoms more obviously to scleroderma.

A feature which usually makes a diagnosis of scleroderma more likely is the beginning of diffuse swelling in the fingers and, less commonly, in the toes. The whole digit swells, not only the region right around the joints; the hand becomes stiff, less successful in its design function of gripping, and difficult to make into a fist. Fairly rapidly thereafter, this edematous, or swollen, face of the disease begins to be superseded by more of a scarification process involving the building up of collagen layers and a resultant thickening of the skin. Various terms such as "hidebound," "leathery," or "contraction of the skin" have been applied to this diffuse thickening process. Sometimes patients also experience calcinosis, the development of small, white subcutaneous lumps, similar in appearance to the pustules of poison ivy.

By the time the collagen build-up has moved to a region closer than the dorsum of hand or wrist, ascending up the extremities and getting closer to the trunk, a diagnosis of scleroderma becomes inescapable.

At this juncture, the physician is faced with a very important decision in differentiating between the two common forms of the disease. In diffuse scleroderma, the more serious kind, the scarification or hardening process begins not only to extend upward along the limbs, but also rapidly involves the trunk, neck, face, and the entirety of the body's skin. In addition, at this stage there are early signs of other organ damage (people often forget that the skin is an organ, too), evidence that the disease is progressing with equal or even more devastating effects inside the body beyond the patient's and physician's view. The esophagus, the gastrointestinal tract, the heart, and the lungs are very frequently involved. Bones, equally deprived of proper blood flow, can become brittle and prone to easy fracture.

The hardening of the skin leads to functional abnormalities in all of these tissues. Typically, for example, when the gastrointestinal system becomes scarified, it loses its natural motility, and food contents and liquids tend to back up almost as though the body is making a dam for the forward propulsion of these nutrients. Heartburn is common, along with swings between chronic constipation and diarrhea. Reduced blood flow can cause dizziness, which in turn can result in serious falls. Swallowing becomes difficult and, eventually for some, impossible. The heart no longer pumps blood effectively, and when the disease attacks the lungs the scarring leads to stiffening, noncompliance, and problems in ventilation and moving air. Also, oxygen is less readily available to the blood because of the thickening of the airways lining the lung. These are among the principal reasons why diffuse scleroderma, when unchecked, leads most frequently to death.

A milder systemic form of scleroderma is CREST syndrome, in which five of these symptoms occur at once: Calcinosis, Raynaud's phenomenon, Esophageal dysfunction, Sclerodactyly, and Telangiectasia. Survival rates for CREST patients are significantly higher than with other diffuse forms.

Many times a diagnosis of diffuse or systemic scleroderma (SSc) can be supported by a relatively new autoantibody test designated antitopoisomerase antibody reactivity; the old term for this test was the anti-Scl-70 test.

In the more benign, limited form of scleroderma, the process seems to stop after a while, so the thickening of the skin may reach about as far as the elbows without going any further, and the internal organs are involved less frequently. One form, morphea, is characterized by discolored patches over the whole body. Another, called linear scleroderma, presents in bands of heavy scarring which can actually extend into the structure of the bones. Unlike most other forms, this usually first appears in children under ten. The extreme resulting disfigurement is described as "a strike of the sword" or *en coup de sabre*. A diagnosis of limited scleroderma in any of these forms gains additional support if another autoantibody—the anti-centromere antibody—is detected in the patient's serum.

In either its systemic or limited forms, the exact cause and etiology of scleroderma continue to elude positive identification, despite decades of investigation. There is mounting evidence that it involves an infection somewhere in the process, and for several years a number of researchers have claimed to identify organisms that looked like the tuberculosis germ in skin tissues from patients with the disease. More recent work has raised the possibility of an abnormality in the immune system, while researchers funded by the Scleroderma Research Foundation speculate that the fibrosis "may be a self-sustaining process built on an autocrine loop—a positive feedback cycle which requires no immunologic input." If that latter view proves correct, it would explain why the immune modifiers tested so frequently against scleroderma have led inevitably to disappointment.

The disappointment is understandable. Regardless of how scleroderma begins, what happens next certainly *looks like* a by-product of autoimmune-based reactivity, the process occurring when the body's immune system, which is designed to provide protection from maladies such as cancer or invasions by infectious organisms, goes awry and begins to attack its own tissues.

In scleroderma, the tissues that seem particularly vulnerable to such attack include the skin and largely collagen-containing areas of the body such as the heart, lungs, and gastrointestinal tract. Collagen is a major structural protein, a kind of natural glue that holds together everything from the bones to the skin. It is a paradox of the disease that not only is collagen-containing tissue frequently subjected to inflammation and eventual damage, but the process is also accompanied by increased collagen deposition far in excess of the body's needs. This overproduction accounts for the hardening and scarification, and is the central feature of the scleroderma (hard skin) process.

An inevitable corollary to the thickening process in scleroderma is an abnormality in the vascular system. The blood vessels begin to decrease, not only in number but also in size or caliber. This relates to the scarring process, but at the moment nobody is sure which is the chicken and which is the egg. Possibly the vascular abnormality and the resulting diminishment in the flow of blood to the tissues are the cause of the collagen build-up. Conversely, the blood vessel deprivation may simply result from the increased hardening of the skin, a process in which the accumulating collagen deposition squeezes out the blood vessels and cuts off the blood supply to the organ structure.

In terms of treatment, scleroderma has been among the most frustrating of all connective tissue diseases. Even though there are still no sure-fire cures for any of the rheumatic illnesses, clinical trials of new treatment modalities such as the tetracycline class of antibiotics are offering new relief for an increasing percentage of patients with rheumatoid arthritis, lupus, even disorders such as fibromyalgia. Up to the time of the Boston study, the same could not be said of scleroderma. It has been gravely discouraging to sufferers and physicians alike that despite decades of testing and retesting, not a single therapy proposed for scleroderma has withstood the scrutiny of carefully controlled clinical trials.

Although penicillamine has been shown in placebo-controlled tests to lack any detectable benefit for scleroderma, in the absence of a viable alternative—and perhaps because some physicians would rather offer something they know won't work than admit they have nothing at all—it is still frequently prescribed.

Other treatments that have been selected for trials in this disease have similarly failed or, if they have appeared to hint at some small benefit, have proven to be too toxic for widespread application. A while back, for example, based on its reported utility in rheumatoid arthritis, researchers tried total lymphoid irradiation, a treatment designed to suppress an abnormally reactive—or overly excited—immune system in a way analogous to its proven utility in the treatment of lymphoid malignancies such as Hodgkin's disease. An extremely drastic treatment, it was found to be totally ineffective in the treatment of scleroderma.

More recently, two other quite toxic drugs may or may not have shown minimal usefulness in scleroderma: cyclophosphamide and cyclosporin. But again, these are drugs designed either to treat malignancies or to preserve transplants of such organs as liver, heart, or kidneys, and they both carry totally unacceptable risk-benefit ratios for widespread implementation with scleroderma.

Although kidney failure is relatively uncommon in scleroderma, patients who have been educated by their doctors or who have made the effort to learn about their disease from other sources are aware— and constantly in fear—that almost without warning it can lead to rapid, severe renal failure. When it happens, very often the only advance notice is the onset of a severe headache and cessation of normal urine flow, both concomitant with an extreme rise in blood pressure to the dangerously high levels that can lead to a stroke.

In the past, this renal failure has been considered to be irreversible, and unless patients received a donor kidney or promptly were placed on dialysis, the process was inevitably lethal. Fortunately, within the last decade or so, drugs called angiotensin-converting enzymes (ACE) inhibitors have been proven capable of reversing this event. Renal failure is still extremely dangerous and can be highly injurious even when the ACE inhibitors work; many patients are left with a degree of kidney damage that is irreversible and tends to produce additional morbidity in the following months or years.

Scleroderma doesn't always follow the same path or pace and doesn't always reach the same result, either in the ultimate extent of damage or incidence of death. Sometimes it takes a slow, protracted, relatively indolent course, fortunately allowing the body to adapt somewhat and giving the patient time to get used to the progressive physical impairment and dysfunction as well as making the psychological adjustments necessary to get the most out of his or her life despite the disease—sometimes for years or even decades of fairly functional and vital life.

On the other hand, it is impossible to predict the subset of perhaps a third to a half of all patients with diffuse scleroderma where the process takes on an almost malignant character. The pace is rapid, deterioration is dramatic, and within just a few months to a year or two the amount of scarring in the skin and internal organs is insurmountable to maintain any degree of functioning, and the patient rapidly approaches death. The heart may fail, and the lungs can either fail or be overwhelmed by bacterial organisms, leading to a fatal pneumonia. Probably the majority of scleroderma-related deaths are associated with lung damage or pneumonia, while some 20 percent each are due to failure of the heart or kidneys.

Other times, quite paradoxically and again unpredictably, the patient can begin with an accelerated disease process only to have it plateau for a number of months or years and even sometimes to demonstrate a degree of reversal or restoration of normalcy.

Although this happens only seldom, the scleroderma can start off very rapidly, then the symptoms decline; the skin begins to soften, there may even be a degree of improvement in the functioning of the lungs, swelling will improve, and constipation becomes less of a problem. In those rare instances, the disease starts off with a frightening vengeance, only to be seemingly thwarted by unknown body mechanisms, independent of any kind of treatment.

There are no surrogate markers or predictors for what kind of course the patient is apt to take.

It is important early in the course of Raynaud's phenomenon for the physician to differentiate that not uncommon event from the more serious process which graduates into scleroderma. Any time a patient develops Raynaud's, which occurs with far greater frequency in young women, the patient and the doctor must both be vigilant to the fact that in the first year or two the small minority of cases wind up as something far worse. Though Raynaud's deteriorates into scleroderma only rarely, the fact that it can occur at all produces a certain amount of psychological stress on the knowledgeable patient and the appropriately vigilant physician. (Even in cases where it doesn't wind up as scleroderma, the Raynaud's sufferer isn't necessarily off the hook. The condition can also serve as a kind of bellwether for lupus and can sometimes be a precursor of rheumatoid arthritis.)

Another common but not inevitable characteristic of scleroderma is that the skin can break down, particularly in the fingers, to leave ulcers on the outside joints which, because of the scarring and the restricted blood supply to the region, are notoriously resistant to healing. These ulcers in turn can become infected, a result that frequently can lead to death through septicemia.

Among the family of rheumatic or connective tissue diseases, scleroderma probably is psychologically the most devastating. It's true that rheumatoid arthritis can be a serious crippler, but it reaches that extreme form in less than 30 percent of all cases. More importantly, most rheumatoid arthritis patients now are aware that effective treatment is finally available, and even if crippling does eventually occur, it becomes problematical in the majority of such cases only after several years or even decades of involvement. And while rheumatoid arthritis is known to be life-shortening, in relatively rare instances does it prove to be fatal.

By contrast, scleroderma can be radically disfiguring as well as severely crippling and the source of terrible pain. Patients know the subsequent course of their disease is unpredictable, and if they manage to overcome their own fears and the frequent reticence of their physician in order to really learn about it, then they become aware that it is not responsive to any currently available treatment and they don't have much to look forward to. As they progress through the disease, they often feel as though they are being moved closer and closer to the abyss.

These factors are hard enough, but there is one other element that adds to the psychological burden, and that is isolation. In most cases, patients who learn they are suffering from a difficult or potentially devastating disease can find some comfort in the encouragement and experience of others who are going through the same trial. There are all kinds of support groups for patients with asthma, diabetes, cancer, and the various forms of arthritis, but that is very rarely the case with scleroderma.

Many times the patient knows next to nothing about the disease, including the two-to-one probability that the diffuse form, which afflicts nearly half of them, will result in death within a decade. In most cases, the physicians making the diagnosis or treating the scleroderma must acknowledge that their experience is extremely limited, based on its rarity and the unlikelihood that they would have encountered it previously. It may sound like a large number if we accept the conservative estimate that 350,000 Americans suffer from scleroderma, but if each of them were to be treated by a different physician, that would still leave two-thirds of the doctors in America who might never lay eyes on a single patient with the disease. Obviously, the number who have never seen it is several times higher.

Not that the advanced form, once encountered, is easy to forget. Scleroderma is a disease with major cosmetic implications. Beyond a certain point, people suffering from it cannot hide the fact that something terrible is happening to their bodies. Patients frequently tell their doctors in the initial stages that it is a heck of a way to get rid of wrinkles, but the remark is a form of gallows humor that says far more about their feeling of apartness and the entirely rational fear of what is yet to come.

Later, as eyebrows disappear and hairlines recede, as the mouth shrinks and reshapes into a ragged rim that no longer closes against the exposed teeth, the wrinkle-free condition can evolve into the leathery hardness of a polished saddle. Body weight can decline precipitously, and fingers can contract downward toward the palms in the form of rigid claws. The face, at last incapable of natural expression and retaining little of its owner's original identity, assumes the macabre and soulless serenity of a death mask.

Given the sense of isolation resulting from its rarity, its painful, uncertain course, and the frightened or distancing response it often produces from others, the afflicted patient can reasonably be led to ask, "Why me? Why have I been so set apart?"

The answer doesn't appear to lie in any kind of heredity pattern, so the patient can't blame his or her genes. No one has any provable theory for how it is transmitted, although the Allegheny County study may offer the subtlest hint that there is an environmental factor. It's pretty certain you can't catch it from smoking, drinking, staying up late, or dancing on Sundays, so the patient is deprived of both the chance to correct errant behavior and any solace to be found in self-recrimination.

Indeed, "Why me?" It is at the same time the most poignant and most relevant question anyone can ask about this terrible disease.

## CHAPTER THREE

# Onset

In June of 1956, near the start of her vacation between high school and college, Pat Stubner met her future husband on a blind date while at her family's summer home in Buffalo, New York. Bill Ganger was four years older than Pat, a muscular, handsome twenty-two, recently out of the army and working in construction. They were inseparable through that summer, and in the fall when she started at Ohio State in Columbus, he came down to visit her about once a quarter. By then, it was obvious that things were getting serious.

Because of that, Pat began thinking about what problems the difference in their educations could cause later if they decided to make the relationship permanent, and with characteristic straightforwardness she told Bill she wouldn't marry him unless he went to college too. So he started at Ohio State on the G.I. Bill, working at paying jobs on nights and weekends. They were married in Pat's junior year, when she was twenty and Bill was twenty-four. Two years later, when Pat graduated and their first child was born, Bill began to feel lost in the crowd at Ohio State and transferred to a smaller city college to finish his degree requirements.

Most of Pat's education was toward the goal of becoming a teacher, but when their daughter Chris came along she decided she was happy being a housewife and mother, so she hung her liberal arts degree over the washing machine and cheerfully gave up any thoughts of a career. Meanwhile, Bill had started working at the campus bar to support the family and help with tuition. In 1962, shortly after he graduated with a degree in industrial management, Bill told Pat that the owner had decided to move to Colorado and had offered to sell him the bar.

It was a hard decision, and when visiting with their families back in Buffalo, the young couple took many a long walk on the shore of Lake Erie, pondering their future. Most of Pat's family had been self-employed, and she knew the risks and drawbacks in Bill striking out on his own. In addition, she felt sure that if Bill went ahead it would be a lifetime commitment, that after becoming his own boss he probably would find it nearly impossible to change his mind later and go to work for someone else. They balanced the freedom and excitement of independence against what appeared in those days to be the security of a corporate career with a steady salary and a guaranteed pension. By the time they returned to Columbus, Bill's optimism had prevailed over Pat's more cautious conservatism, and he told his boss they had decided to take the gamble.

From a business viewpoint, it was a safe decision. The bar was right across the street from an arena that attracted tens of thousands of people to a variety of sports events, and most of the regular patrons were an older crowd from the nearby dental school, a steady clientele less prone to the wildness typical at other college hangouts. But thirteen years later, after a third of a lifetime of seven-day weeks and arriving home from his job at two o'clock in the morning, Bill decided it was time to look at some other line of work.

He tried running a travel agency for a while, but he kept thinking of something that had happened in the last few months he owned the bar, suspecting it represented an opportunity with even greater promise.

It started with his running out of some forms he used for inventory control. It was a simple one-page sheet, and Bill didn't get around to doing anything about it until the supply had dwindled down to nearly the final copy. When he brought that last page to the nearest printer, an old-timer who had been in the business for years, he was told the cost would be forty-seven dollars and delivery wouldn't be for a week. He needed it right away, so the next stop was at a storefront with a sign above the door that said "Quick Printing." There he was told the job would be ready the following day, at half the price, and Bill could keep the scraps.

On his way home and for months afterward, he found himself turning over the experience in his mind. He had recognized instantly that the printing industry was undergoing a revolution, and he couldn't free himself of the sense that during this period of rapid change, with every day that passed he was missing another chance to improve his life.

When Bill and Pat Ganger opened their own quick-printing shop in 1975, they were painfully aware how little either of them knew about their new business. By mostly trial and error they learned where to buy paper, which end of the machine to feed it into, and how to trim, collate, fold, and bind the resulting product. The first time they had to print envelopes, with Bill standing at one end of the machine and Pat at the other they successively tried each of the myriad knobs, buttons, and switches until they hit on the combination that worked. "Okay," Bill told Pat when the first envelope finally zipped through successfully, "send down the rest." Slowly and steadily, the business grew in size and profits.

Seven years into their printing venture, in the fall of 1982, Pat sprained an ankle at their newly purchased summer home on Pelee Island in Lake Erie. She slipped off a log, and although it was not a major event at the time, it seemed to take forever to heal. It wasn't until early the following winter that things got bad enough that the Gangers realized they were dealing with something more than the protracted aftermath of the summertime mishap. In late December, still not free of the pain of her injury, Pat noticed something new and apparently unrelated to the problem with her ankle: a pins-and-needles sensation in her hands when she woke up in the morning. At first she thought it was from her hands "going to sleep" because she had been lying on them during the night, but when the feeling recurred on a regular basis, sometimes even before she went to bed, she began to realize something else might be going on.

A short time later, her right leg started to swell from the knee down. Like the tingling hands, the swelling was uncomfortable, but this time the symptom was something that could be clearly seen by others, so she decided to show it to their local doctor. He was an old family practitioner just getting ready to retire, and the examination was brief. After drawing some blood and the most casual inspection, he told

Pat not to give it another thought; lots of women her age were likely to swell up for no reason at all. He wrote out a prescription for a diuretic and told her to come back in a month if the edema persisted. Back home, Pat said to Bill, half in jest, "I'm beginning to think I'm in trouble."

The blood test was normal, but the diuretic didn't have any effect at all on the swelling. In fact, within two weeks the same condition appeared in her other leg and Pat called back to say she was only getting worse.

During her second examination the doctor drew blood again, only this time he ordered some of the standard tests for rheumatic disease. He later called to report that her antinuclear antibody (ANA) reading was a slightly elevated 200, and the sedimentation rate was in the high normal range at around 10. Pat didn't know what either of those terms meant at the time, but she made a note of them for possible future interest. She was right in suspecting she would have reason to refer to them again.

The family doctor said there was nothing to worry about, but just to be on the safe side he was going to send her to an internist. Another series of tests was performed, but still nothing definitive showed up in her blood. Neither she nor either of the doctors had yet made a connection between the tingling in her hands and the swollen legs, but Pat was hardly reassured by the lack of a diagnosis. This time when she went home, she told Bill she thought there was something seriously wrong going on in her body, and they were just waiting for it to come out.

During subsequent visits to the internist, although no one had yet put a specific name to her problem, for the first time she heard the term "connective tissue disease." When she repeated it to Bill, he asked what it meant and she said she didn't know. The next day, he went to the library at Ohio State Medical School to see what he could learn about it.

Pat, meanwhile, was in a kind of never-never land, worn out and depressed by the rigors of an unspecified illness, growing resentful at the lack of serious sympathy that she felt sure this same condition would receive, especially at home, if only it had a name. She knew she wasn't really sick enough to take to her bed, and she agreed with Bill that she shouldn't give in to it. But sometimes his insistence that she keep working, that she try to live a normal life, felt a bit like callousness or indifference. He obviously cared deeply about what was happening to her, but he was a fighter and his response was different from what she thought she wanted. Some nights, when he returned from the medical school library with new data on connective tissues and the various diseases under that broad heading, she would find herself thinking that the information, possibly even irrelevant to her illness, was nowhere nearly as soothing as sympathy.

Casting his diagnostic net in progressively wider arcs, the internist increased the scope of the tests. An ENG, or electroneurograph, determined that there was no detectable injury or disease peripheral to the nerves. Although this test involves a kind of mapping of the neural system through a series of pinpricks and is normally considered to be moderately uncomfortable, the swelling was so severe that until the doctor accidentally burst a capillary on her upper thigh, Pat had felt nothing and was unaware even that the procedure involved the puncturing of her skin.

A venogram, designed to reveal thromboses or obstructions in the veins through the use of injected dyes, went the same way. Unable to find a vein in her leg or foot, the doctor ordered a large bucket-like container to be filled with hot water to reduce the swelling enough to find a point of entry for the needle.

A wide variety of new blood work was ordered, including a CPK, or creatinine phosphokinase test, in a futile search for evidence of some injury to the muscles of the heart, skeleton, or brain.

Along the way, Pat was beginning to resent the way the internist treated the product of their joint efforts. He wouldn't give her numbers and was extremely guarded with test results, dismissing her queries with remarks like, "Well, it's not bad considering . . ."

"Considering what?" she would ask, but he always parried with a digression or a shrug. He made it clear that he didn't like being asked questions—not, she guessed, because he was threatened by a challenge, but because he believed the only aspect of this process to which the patient had any legitimate claim was a good clinical result. Obviously the doctor's medical knowledge and whatever insights they developed along the way were his alone.

When one day the doctor mentioned connective tissue disease again, Pat asked him what that meant.

"Well, like lupus or scleroderma."

Pat had never heard of either one, and asked what they were.

He appeared to weigh the value of making an effort, then apparently decided against it, waving the subject shut with a gesture of dismissal. "They're hard to explain."

"Can you try?" she persisted, smiling hopefully.

He just smiled back and said, "No."

Chafing at the lack of progress and the growing sense that no one, including the internist, was really taking responsibility for her case, Pat and Bill decided to begin calling other specialists; if they couldn't identify what was the matter with her, at least they could eliminate some of the obvious possibilities. Typically the appointments were spaced at two-week intervals because that was how long it took to get an open date. Even with insurance there were limits to how much they could spend, so they decided to schedule them in a series rather than all at the same time.

A major exception was the referral to a dermatologist at the local medical school that involved a much longer wait because the doctor was so well-known. Pat became impatient. The swelling obviously involved her skin, and she reasoned the dermatologist should be at the start of the referral chain rather than so much further down the line. So she decided to jump the gun.

By this time, the swelling wasn't the only problem; more ominously, the skin in the vicinity of the sprain was beginning to tighten, almost as though her body was exchanging the normal, healthy tissue there for a hard, slick, sickly white shell. She looked up dermatology in the Yellow Pages, found a physician near where she lived, and scheduled an office visit for the end of that week. She still intended to keep the other appointment much later, but this might offer her a useful preview.

The dermatologist was a quiet, kindly man, perhaps nearing seventy, and he examined her legs with a great deal of interest. Pat had told him her situation with the other doctors, and that she was just looking for another opinion in advance of her meeting with the specialist at the medical school. "Your skin looks like paraffin," he said, glancing up at her as though for affirmation.

Pat decided it was a question, so she looked at her legs and agreed it did.

He left the examination room for a moment, then returned from his office with a heavy medical tome which he placed on the table where she was sitting. He leafed through to the back, then pointed to a section of dense type. "'The skin takes on a paraffin-like appearance,'" he read aloud. He scanned a few more lines in silence, then closed the book without further comment. "I haven't seen a case before," he said quietly, "but it looks to me like scleroderma."

This time Pat recognized the term, although she still knew nothing more about the disease than when it was mentioned in casual speculation a few days before by her internist. She nodded and repeated "Scleroderma," as though making the word her own. From the way the dermatologist said it, scleroderma sounded no more ominous than eczema or psoriasis, and she didn't even bother asking him how to spell it.

The doctor left her alone to put on her stockings, and she didn't see him again until she got to the front desk and asked for her bill. The receptionist told her there was no charge, and Pat turned in bewilderment to the doctor.

"Because I didn't do anything for you," he said, waving aside her protests. "I just gave you an opinion, and I'm not going to charge you."

She thanked him profusely, and he replied with a smile and a pat on the shoulder as he opened the door, "I wish you well."

In the years since then, Pat would remember him with gratitude for his warmth and generosity—and with a nagging, never-answered question in her mind about whether he had decided not to charge her because he had read the rest of that passage in the book and knew what lay ahead.

In the several weeks that followed that visit, no one mentioned scleroderma to Pat again. The succession of specialists—eventually nine of them—continued on. The internist, who knew what she was doing, suggested she enter the hospital for a couple of days so all the tests could be done at once. Pat refused on the grounds she was too busy, but that and the money weren't the only reasons. Entering the hospital even for a diagnosis would have been a form of surrender to whatever it was that was trying to bring her down. She was determined to fight it on her feet.

The Gangers were learning to fight back in other ways as well. One doctor gave Pat some test results in a sealed envelope addressed to the internist who ordered them, and as she drove across town between the two offices, she kept glancing down at the secret message on the seat beside her and realized that she was becoming extremely angry. She detoured to the print shop and showed the envelope to Bill. "These are tests of *my* blood, taken from *my* body, paid with *my* money, for a disease that nobody can identify, and I'm not even allowed to look at them."

Bill took the envelope from her hand and examined it briefly on the light table where he was pasting up a layout. It was a No. 10 Universal in 24# white, and the cornercard was a simple name and address, with no logo, set in black New Times Roman. "You've got a point," he said, tearing open the flap. They then photocopied the contents, set new type for the cornercard, cranked up the press, and less than five minutes later were resealing the report in a new envelope indistinguishable from the original.

For all that effort, the only thing they learned was the name of one more disease she didn't have, with no new insights to the one she did.

The internist's next referral was to a neurologist who tapped her knees and ankles with a rubber hammer and then ran some small wires down her legs and asked if she could feel them. When he finished, he said he said he didn't think the problem originated with her nerves, adding that he saw no reason to do a proposed biopsy.

Because this doctor appeared willing to communicate, Pat shared with him that she had been out of town for a short time, and the swelling had substantially decreased during that period. "It got worse when I returned."

He asked her where she worked, and when she said a print shop, he asked if that involved exposure to a lot of chemicals. She said it did.

"That could be the connection," he said. "Can you go away again, and see what happens?"

By then it was well into spring, and Pat decided to take a six-week sabbatical on Pelee Island. She opened their house on the shore, and carefully planned every day so that it included a balanced diet, plenty of rest, and a reasonable amount of exercise, starting with a walk.

In the first few days, the walk was the biggest challenge. She could barely go six hundred feet along the beach before she found herself sitting down heavily on a log, overwhelmed with fatigue and fighting to recover her failing breath. If she saw something of interest by the water's edge, she didn't have the energy to bend down to examine it or pick it up. By the end of her six-week vacation both her stamina and flexibility had improved measurably. But almost as soon as she got back to Columbus, her legs began to swell again and the fatigue was as bad as ever.

She stayed at home for a few days but didn't get any better. The next test was the house. Pat stayed with her mother for a week and continued to keep away from the print shop, but the change in routine produced no effect on her condition. Neither they nor the doctor were able to come up with an environmental combination that duplicated or explained the improvement she found during her solitary vacation on Pelee Island.

Frustrated by a growing sense of deadlock with her internist, in rapid succession Pat visited a dermatologist, a gynecologist, and an allergist. She and Bill had decided that if no one could identify her problem, at least they could eliminate a number of things it wasn't. The new strategy proved to be no more productive than the old.

They both felt they had hit bottom when she finally kept the appointment with the popular dermatologist at the local teaching hospital. He appeared distracted throughout the interview, and at first they thought it was a part of his obvious shyness. When either Pat or Bill attempted eye contact, he had a habit of studying the floor or looking down at his desk as though searching for an answer, but it was soon apparent that he had no such difficulty when talking about her condition with the five students who were sitting in on the examination. Even when Pat asked him a direct question, he would look at the students rather than at her when he answered, demonstrating a level of empathy and engagement more appropriate to a cadaver or an anatomist's dummy. The focus of his interest soon narrowed to an insistence that they'd never get to the true nature of her disease unless Pat permitted him to perform a biopsy of the tissue on her hand.

She refused outright. The dermatologist asked her a second time and then a third, but she wouldn't budge. Two previous doctors had warned her against just that procedure, one on the grounds that there were too many tendons and nerves beneath the swelling to avoid with certainty the risk of causing permanent damage, and the other because there was no apparent disease involvement in her hands at that point, and unless the biopsy disclosed specific activity it would be unproductive. But the real reason for her refusal was that the situation reminded her in many ways of the incident with the sealed envelope. She was paying the doctor for a visit, only to find herself excluded from the process. Instead of providing any form of treatment, offering insights or sharing in his knowledge of the possibilities, the doctor had used her almost exclusively as a teaching tool for the benefit of his students.

The dermatologist partially redeemed himself two weeks later when he called to ask Pat how she was doing, but he was still obviously stymied by her case and he offered no suggestion for what either of them might try next. Anyway, by then she had traveled on through the system and was in the hands of an allergist.

As had most of the other doctors, the allergist said he wanted to begin with a brief physical. Apparently concerned that Pat might think such a rudimentary procedure was beside the point of her visit, he explained that sometimes doctors overlook the obvious, adding almost apologetically, "I don't want to get burned." She told him she understood, and was used to it.

It was not the allergist, however, who performed the examination. He left the room and a younger man—perhaps a medical student or a physician's assistant—came in and after a few brief preliminaries he started listening to her heart with a stethoscope. He listened and listened, so intent on his task that Pat began to wonder what he thought he was hearing. After a few minutes of intense concentration, he excused himself and left the room. The allergist then returned alone and told Pat he was referring her to a cardiologist. "Set a date and then go home and get into bed," he said, "and stay there until your appointment."

Despite Pat's direct questions, neither the doctor nor his associate offered any clue to what the problem might be, so she and Bill obediently climbed into their car and drove the few blocks to the address on the referral slip.

It was early May, just before the annual running of the Kentucky Derby, and the walls of the cardiologist's office were covered with pictures of thoroughbred horses. The receptionist told them the nearest available date was two weeks away. Although they knew by then that two weeks was about the standard wait for a first appointment in their long chain of referrals, this time Bill balked at the possibility that Pat would have to spend the next two weeks in bed for no better reason, for all he knew, than that the cardiologist was at Churchill Downs watching a horse race. When he explained that they had been told it was urgent, the receptionist excused herself to go down the hall for a brief conference with the doctor, then returned and said he would see Pat the following day.

That night Pat lay in bed and wondered what desperate new turn her situation had taken that the allergist considered her to be at such risk. The next afternoon, however, those anxieties vanished almost as soon as she walked into the cardiologist's office. The new doctor surveyed her as he shook her hand, and he made no attempt to hide an expression of growing puzzlement. "You don't have a heart problem," he told her. "I can tell just by looking at you."

As welcome as those words were, Pat quickly agreed to submit to the few brief tests the cardiologist proposed to confirm his evaluation. The EKG was normal, and so was the echocardiogram subsequently performed at the local hospital. Pat asked again what it was the allergist and his associate had heard that they thought was so serious.

"You have a functional heart murmur," the doctor said. "So do millions of other Americans, and it doesn't mean a thing." The problem, he explained, was that when a physician hears a murmur in a patient whose legs are as swollen as Pat's, that can be an indicator that the heart isn't doing its job. In her case her arms were swollen too, if not as badly, her complexion was good, and except for the murmur she showed none of the other classic signs of heart disease. Because the arms are above the heart, he finished, it seemed immediately likely to a cardiologist, if not to an allergist, that the swelling in either set of limbs had nothing to do with the murmur.

The Gangers paid the cardiologist $360, most of which was for the tests, but when Pat received a bill from the allergist for another sixty dollars, she called his office and said she was rejecting it. Although she had no doubt that the allergist was a very caring doctor and she liked him personally, the referral to the cardiologist had been expensive and unnecessary. The real problem was that the allergist hadn't done anything related to the reason she went to him. He didn't run a single test, and she still had no more idea after her visit whether her problem was related to an allergy.

The reason for the visit to the gynecologist, who came next, was to eliminate the possibility of an imbalance in her hormone levels. After an examination and some blood tests which eliminated that possibility and gave no hint to the cause of her problem, she made an appointment with her ophthalmologist.

She had seen the eye doctor some months earlier because of a cataract which had developed long before the accident on Pelee Island. At the outset it had been a mildly annoying haze across one eye and they had agreed to wait and see how it developed. Now the doctor looked at it briefly and told Pat he thought it was time they consider surgery. She answered that she wanted to wait, that she had other problems she felt she needed to deal with first, and she showed him the swelling in her legs and arms. He glanced briefly at her skin and said, "It looks like connective tissue disease." She was amazed. How was an ophthalmologist able to identify a condition that had eluded so many other specialists?

That May, more than five months after she saw her first doctor for the problem that had started in her legs, Pat happened to go to a local family practitioner, an osteopath, for a routine stomach upset. In passing, she mentioned the chain of events that had begun on Pelee Island the year before. In addition to his general practice he specialized in sports medicine, and he quickly pointed out that he was an unlikely source for a solution. But he asked Pat who was coordinating all the data she was developing from all the other specialists she had visited, and when she told him no one, he volunteered for the job.

Osteopaths tend to take a holistic view, looking at a patient as a whole person rather than focusing narrowly or exclusively on an area of specialization, and Pat quickly accepted the offer. The doctor wrote to all the previous physicians and in short order he had collected a fat folder on her medical odyssey. One of the great frustrations throughout Pat's experience with the other doctors had been their general unwillingness to explain or even share with her the data they had developed about her condition. The osteopath made it clear at the outset that would no longer be the case. "This is your file, and everything in it belongs to you," he said. "It's yours to read anytime you want, and if there are any parts of it you don't understand, just ask."

Paradoxically, the doctors who wrote the longest, most detailed responses were the ones who had seen Pat the fewest times. The only area in which they were in full agreement was that it was a fascinating, perplexing case. Most surprising to Pat was how many of their reports included small errors, such as the physician who recalled giving her a cortisone shot in the shoulder when in fact it had been in her hip.

The family practitioner also had an assignment for Pat. He told her to write down all of the changes that had taken place in her body since the problem had begun. By then it was nearly a year since the sprained ankle on Pelee, but most of the changes on the lined yellow fourteen-inch legal sheet which she handed him on her next visit had taken place in just the past five or six months, since her visit to the first doctor in December.

In addition to the swelling in her legs and then her arms, several little islands of shiny skin had started to appear on other parts of her body, especially across her chest and on the backs of her hands. For most of her lifetime she had had unusually soft fingernails, so flexible that when she was in high school and had let the nail on her pinkie grow out, she had been able to fold it across the top of the finger without breaking it. Now her nails had all become much thicker, less pliant, and more prone to chipping. She had started losing her hair, and even when she was careful in her grooming, there were broken tangles in her comb and on her brush. As the skin on her body appeared to tighten, she was finding it more and more difficult to bend over, to get out of a deep chair, to enter or exit a car.

She had also begun to notice changes in the two outside fingers on her right hand. They were losing their suppleness, becoming awkward to use in such familiar tasks as typing and even washing her face. They no longer assumed the usual easy alignment with the rest of her fingers when the hand was at rest but were starting to contract inward toward the palm, as though curling around an invisible object.

The osteopath looked at the list and suggested an arthritis profile, but the results were far from definitive. He next ran several of the tests she originally had hoped to get from the allergist, and there were no major revelations there either. However, they did discover a reaction to some of the chemicals she had worked with on a regular basis over the past several years at the print shop. The allergic response wasn't strong enough to explain all her other symptoms, but Pat wondered if perhaps the accumulated chemicals had lowered her resistance or in some similar way had acted as a kind of enabler to the events that followed her ankle sprain.

By the end of the summer, at a loss for any other avenue of approach, they decided to take a closer look at one of the shiny patches of skin. The osteopath agreed that it could be risky to perform the procedure on her hands or feet, so they settled on the chest. The punch biopsy made a small indentation about the size of a .22 caliber bullet hole just a few inches below her clavicle. It also produced the long-sought diagnosis.

When Pat met with the doctor after the results came back from the lab, he handed her the report without comment. By then she was used to his open sharing of all the paperwork in her case, but this time his silence was ominous and she could tell he was disturbed. She looked down at the sheet and read that the analysis had found collagen bundles in the sample tissues. She knew vaguely that collagen was one of the things in the body that help build skin, so she saw no particular significance in the presence of bundles of it in her biopsy. The other word that caught her attention was scleroderma; some months before, it was one of the two examples her internist had offered her of connective tissue disease.

"That's what I've got?" she asked, looking up. "Scleroderma?"

He nodded.

"What is it? What does it mean?"

The doctor said he had never seen a case before, but it was clear that he was trying hard not to dodge the question. He explained that when the report came in he had called an older physician who sometimes acted as his mentor, but he had never seen a case either. He went on to tell her the word means 'hard skin.' It was a very serious disease, and relatively rare. Nobody knew what caused it. There were several possible treatments and sometimes they helped, but none was considered a cure.

"So what happens," Pat asked, "if it can't be cured? Can it be fatal?"

The doctor looked down at his desk for an answer, then met her eyes again. "I just don't know that much about it," he said, then added, "But—sometimes, apparently, yes."

She sat back in her chair. For a moment it seemed as if the skin of her swollen legs and arms, as well as the small, shiny patches that were now starting to bind her chest and torso, had noticeably tightened in response to the naming of her disease.

## CHAPTER FOUR

# The Infectious Theory

The modern history of scleroderma—at least *this* modern history—begins in the late 1930s at the Rockefeller Institute, with two of Albert Sabin's mice. Sabin was studying a central nervous system disease called toxoplasmosis, one of the early steps in his quarter-century quest to develop a vaccine against the worldwide scourge of poliomyelitis, or infantile paralysis. At the time of this story he was only thirty-two, and relatively unknown.

The first mouse was sacrificed for a laboratory experiment in which Sabin cultured the dead rodent's brain. Looking for infectious agents, he smeared the culture and tried to stain it. At first he couldn't see any change at all, but in taking a closer look, he thought he detected a very slight clouding of the media, which suggested that something extremely ephemeral, something almost not there, might be hiding in his sample. He ran a further series of tests and determined that the cloud was caused by an L-form, a class of germs thought in those days to be comprised entirely of new phases of bacteria, and which took their name from the Lister Institute in London where they were first described. Some of what were originally called L-forms turned out to be not bacteria at all, but doughnut-shaped organisms about halfway in size between bacteria and viruses. When they were separately identified several years later they were renamed mycoplasmas, a Latin composite of the words for fungus and fluid. In the days before electron microscopy, L-forms or mycoplasmas were still invisible and could be detected only by inference. Sabin pondered his discovery, then drew some of the cloudy fluid into a hypodermic needle and injected it into Mouse #2. Shortly afterward, the second mouse developed a form of inflammatory arthritis.

Sabin walked down the hall and discussed this interesting result with another researcher, a rheumatologist the same age as himself named Thomas McPherson Brown. Like Sabin, Brown was looking for the infectious cause of a major disease, but not polio and not in the central nervous system; Brown's target was rheumatoid arthritis, and his arena was the synovium, the lubricating fluid in the joints. At the same time that Sabin was working with the two mice, after some two hundred attempts Brown had finally succeeded in isolating an L-form, subsequently shown to have been a mycoplasma, from the joint fluid of a human being.

For reasons that are still unknown, the human form of mycoplasma is far more elusive than the mouse version, and much harder to isolate. Brown described his results in a brief article in *Science* in 1939, and again more fully ten years later in *Post Graduate Medicine and Surgery*. No previous researcher had ever found an infectious agent right in the joint, and although Brown's success broke new ground, even a decade later it was predictably greeted with mixed reviews, some hailing it as a milestone in determining an infectious etiology for one of mankind's oldest and most widespread crippling diseases, others dismissing his results as nothing more than a ubiquitous laboratory contaminant. The naysayers gained ground in the months following the *Science* article when no one else was successful in replicating his success. But then, no one else was willing to try more than once or twice before giving up.

Many of the basic discoveries in medicine have been made simply because someone was able to recognize the significance of a widely observed effect. Countless thousands of medical students and laboratory researchers, for example, knew that mold could end an experiment overnight by killing everything they had painstakingly cultured in their petri dishes. Only three such witnesses—Ernest B. Chain, Alexander Fleming, and Howard Florey—thought hard enough about what it meant that they wound up sharing the Nobel prize for the discovery and development of penicillin.

Thomas McPherson Brown had observed such a widely noted effect, although in those days he was not alone in making a connection with its probable cause. He had seen that rheumatoid arthritis can improve for a time in response to the gold and quinine drugs then (as now) commonly used in its treatment, and he theorized that the response meant the disease agent was alive, and therefore infectious. For obvious ethical reasons he couldn't inject a second human with the mycoplasma extracted from someone else's synovium, but to both Brown and Sabin the mouse experiment provided a persuasive model for what would happen if he did.

Paradoxically, the infectious theory of rheumatoid arthritis received a boost from exactly the opposite reaction as well, when patients suffered a serious flareup of their disease in response to medications, especially to antibiotics. When Dr. Louis Dienes and Howard Weinberger published their landmark paper on "Experimental Arthritis: Pleuropneumonia-like Organisms and Their Possible Relation to Articular Disease," which described the L-form as "an invisible, filterable form that may exist after the parent germ disappears," Brown was asked to comment, and he included a discussion of that phenomenon in his 1988 book, *The Road Back*:

> *I reported that we had observed this organism in a number of clinical situations. Seventeen patients representing a wide variety of rheumatic diseases including rheumatoid arthritis, rheumatic spondylitis, chorea, erythema nodosum, and rheumatic fever, were treated with Aureomycin, a tetracycline derivative, because it had an effect on those organisms. . . . [W]hen we started treating these patients with a tetracycline product, they invariably got worse before they started getting better—an event in medicine known as the Jarisch-Herxheimer reaction.*
>
> *This discussion was the first linking in the entire medical literature of the Jarisch-Herxheimer effect with a tetracycline derivative in a rheumatic problem. Presumably the effect was due to the dislodging and breaking up of the mycoplasma and the releasing of antigen to a sensitized field. The effect showed a number of important principles at work. It demonstrated that the disease was a hypersensitive reaction, not to the drug itself but to the toxins that a germ creates in response to the drug's presence. It showed that the germ must indeed be invisible, as Dienes and Weinberger had suggested, because no other germs of such standard types as streptococcus or staphylococcus were isolable. And it opened the way to a chemical attack on the whole area of arthritis and rheumatic disease.*

The door may have been opened, but it would be years before anyone besides Brown walked through it. The *New York Times* devoted an entire page to his breakthrough, but in the absence of verification by other researchers, the excitement was short-lived. Brown returned to Johns Hopkins to become chief resident in medicine. Although the school gave him his own laboratory and a research fellow, he hadn't gotten much further in his study by the start of World War II. Shortly after the Japanese bombing of Pearl Harbor, he received his commission in the military, and in late 1944 he led a small group of researchers in culturing swamp water and searching for a defense against malaria on a recently liberated island in the central Philippines.

On his return to civilian life in 1946, Brown chose against a variety of far more prestigious alternatives to accept a position with the Veterans Administration, based on the opportunity it offered to continue his earlier work, now as head of arthritis research for VA hospitals nationwide. But a different kind of war was brewing on the home front, and he was to become one of its earliest victims.

The cause of the war was cortisone. Extracted from the adrenal cortex by Philip Hench at the Mayo Clinic in the late 1940s, "Compound E," as it was first known, promised to be the most miraculous among the new generation of wonder drugs. It reversed the pain and swelling of rheumatoid arthritis so dramatically that almost overnight it altered the conceptual view of the arthritis mechanism. The question arose of whether arthritis was in the strictest sense a disease at all, but rather a condition, analogous to diabetes, triggered by a kind of metabolic failure. One big difference between the two, however, was known to everyone who had even the most rudimentary laboratory experience in rheumatology: unlike diabetes, in which the body failed to produce the required amount of insulin, patients with the inflammatory forms of arthritis inevitably had far *more* cortisone in their systems than those who were disease-free.

Moreover, in the months following Hench's *tour de force* (for which he later would share the Nobel prize), it became abundantly apparent that too much of a good thing could be very bad indeed. There was no doubt that cortisone, soon commercially formulated as prednisone, deserved its great harvest of acclaim, but in the enormous quantities in which it was often then prescribed, the results were inevitably short-lived and frequently disastrous.

Tom Brown was convinced that the way the new drug worked had nothing to do with the arthritis mechanism, which he still believed was infectious, but rather addressed only the swelling and pain. Clearly this was beneficial, but not if it subverted the search for the true mechanism of arthritis, not if it simply masked symptoms while allowing the disease itself to continue destroying joints, and not if abuses of over-prescription produced new problems far more serious or life-threatening than the ones the drug appeared to solve. He expressed those misgivings, along with an honest appreciation of cortisone's obvious benefits, at the annual meeting of the American Rheumatism Association in 1949.

Brown continued his career as dean of medicine at George Washington University Medical School, then as head of the Arthritis Institute which he founded at the National Hospital for Orthopedics and

Rehabilitation, and he even became a medical consultant to the White House. His clinical practice, based not on politics but on results, continued to prosper. Over the years he treated some ten thousand patients, primarily for rheumatoid arthritis but also with just about every other connective tissue disease known to medicine. He also continued to publish, compiling over one hundred professional papers by the end of his long career. But after 1949 virtually all of his laboratory and clinical research was privately funded. From the time he spoke out at the ARA until the end of his life some four decades later, his access to government funding for research, mediated by his more powerful peers and heavily influenced by the pharmaceutical industry, simply evaporated.

So what does all of this have to do with scleroderma?

Sometime during the 1960s, a woman from Tennessee called Dr. Brown's office for an appointment to treat her rheumatoid arthritis. When she arrived in Washington, Brown was hardly prepared for the gaunt, paraffin-like slickness of her face, the oily whiteness of her fingers, or the ulcerated knuckles of her hands, but he had seen this disease before and immediately recognized its symptoms. She assured him that she already knew she was in the final stages of systemic scleroderma, and that it was incurable. But meanwhile the pain of the arthritis was worsening as well, and she didn't want to deal with it at the same time. He agreed to help, and started her on his customary combination of intravenous and oral antibiotics for the rheumatoid arthritis.

Over the following months, the therapy slowly improved and reversed the ache, swelling, and stiffness of her arthritic joints.

Brown followed her progress with particular interest, and it wasn't just the arthritis he was watching. When she came into his office one day and reported that her scleroderma had started to go away as well, she said she could hardly believe her own words.

Dr. Brown smiled and said he would keep her on the therapy until they got the same result with both diseases. He was nowhere nearly as surprised as she was.

## CHAPTER FIVE

# Connections

Another Southern lady named Katherine Loftis, a housewife from Huntsville, Alabama, found out she had scleroderma in 1976. Typically for that disease, the diagnosis came at the end of a chain of referrals, first from her family doctor to a rheumatologist, and from there to a dermatologist who biopsied a section of her thickened skin. When the last doctor told her the results he looked appropriately somber, saying how sorry he was to be giving her such bad news.

Like most people, before she was told she had it, Katherine wasn't sure if she had ever even heard of the disease. Now, based on the tone of that brief exchange with the skin doctor, she went back to her rheumatologist expecting to hear the worst. His reaction couldn't have been more of a surprise. He told her not to worry about a thing, that they had caught it early, the disease hadn't gotten to the inside of her body yet, and with a little Naprosyn they'd keep it under control and she'd be just fine. Naprosyn is a non-steroidal anti-inflammatory, and the way the rheumatologist talked about the drug and her illness, it didn't sound much more than aspirin for a small headache.

She talked with her family doctor, an internist, right afterwards, and he was appalled. "But that just isn't so," he told her. "It *will* affect your major organs, and it will get progressively worse."

Given the choice, obviously she would far rather have believed the rheumatologist. By then her symptoms had begun to accumulate: slick, unhealthy skin on her fingertips, a progressive thickening and tightening of her face and hands, and a constant, extreme fatigue. Besides, she trusted her internist, and she knew he was telling her the truth. She wondered why the rheumatologist had dismissed her potentially fatal disease with such misleading and inappropriate assurances.

One evening not long after her diagnosis, her husband Lewis read in the newspaper that another rheumatologist, Dr. Thomas McPherson Brown, was coming down from Washington to give a lecture at nearby Huntsville. Both Lewis and Katherine still knew very little about scleroderma and there weren't many places they could go to find out. By then they had learned that it was a connective tissue disease, which meant it was in the same family with the more familiar rheumatoid arthritis and lupus as well as afflictions with such strange, forbidding names as fibromyalgia and spondyloarthropathy. The paper said that Dr. Brown had been very successful in treating rheumatoid arthritis, and Lewis wondered aloud if he might also have some ideas about the disease that was threatening to kill his wife.

Katherine was on the telephone the next morning, repeating Lewis's question to the family doctor. The internist was just as straightforward as he had been about her prognosis. He said it made all the sense in the world, and he was chagrined he hadn't thought of it himself. He offered to telephone the National Hospital on her behalf to discuss her case with Dr. Brown, and when he called her back he said Brown had been very optimistic, that he had successfully treated a few cases already, and that he would be glad to take on Katherine as a patient. The internist forwarded her records to Brown's office in suburban Washington, and three months later, in June of 1978, Katherine Loftis followed them north.

In the interim, and in ironic contrast to the sanguine forecasts of her original rheumatologist, her disease had progressed faster than all expectations. The "butterfly" pattern sometimes associated with scleroderma and far more frequently with lupus had appeared on her face, her cheekbones had risen to new prominence with the drawing back of her tightened skin, and the complexion of her face and hands was alternately a frozen alabaster or a slick, sickly pink. The index and middle fingers of her right hand were so rigid, useless, and lacking in feeling, they could have been made of stone, and her day's supply of energy was exhausted almost before she got out of bed in the morning.

Dr. Brown turned out to be a kindly, deep-chested, good-humored man, apparently in his late fifties, shorter than either of them had expected, with a broad Scottish face, dark but graying hair, a courtly, soft-spoken voice, and a humorous, inquisitive warmth in his dark eyes that was at once pixie-like and deeply intelligent. He cocked his head and looked at Katherine intently when he greeted her, holding her proffered hand in both his own in a way that welcomed and soothed. (A decade later, she learned that the famous Dr. Brown handshake, which seldom lasted more than a few seconds, was a kind of on-the-spot lab test for skin tone and elasticity, circulation, temperature, heart function, and the condition of a patient's nerves, as diagnostically productive as a CAT scan. They would learn far sooner that his age at the time of that first meeting was actually seventy-two.)

When Katherine and Lewis arrived in Arlington it happened to be one of those rare times when Dr. Brown had no other patients at the National Hospital, and that evening after she had settled in they shared a long, reassuring visit in her room. Lewis was particularly concerned at the rapid changes since the diagnosis just three months before, and he opened the conversation by asking Dr. Brown, "What does my wife have to look forward to?"

The unhesitating answer was, "Everything."

Dr. Brown said he had treated a number of scleroderma patients with antibiotic therapy—he estimated seven up to that time—and every one of them had either recovered or was on the road back. He cautioned Katherine and Lewis against expecting too much too soon, however, warning that connective tissue diseases in general were extremely complex, and that it could be months or even several years before she was completely free of its effects.

While Katherine was showering on her third morning at the hospital, barely forty-eight hours after the start of antibiotic therapy, the swelling was so reduced that her rings spontaneously slipped off the fourth finger of her left hand. She could hardly believe it. Dr. Brown was glad to hear the news, but he renewed his caveat: the swelling would return, and it was possible that her condition would actually worsen in the coming six months before it began to improve in a way that lasted.

He was right. Her condition didn't appear to deteriorate in the following months, but it didn't get any better, and as Brown had predicted by the time she returned for her first follow-up visit in December, her scores were all higher than when she began. He was also right about what happened next. By June of 1979, the results had turned around, and the disease parameters measured steadily downward for all of her subsequent semiannual visits.

On her fifth trip to Washington, just thirty-one months after she began treatment, the swelling had all but disappeared, her energy levels were consistently higher, her depression had lifted, and she had no doubt that she was well along the road to recovery. In her fourth year, Dr. Brown came into her hospital room during her December visit and laid out the results from all of her lab tests: for the first time since she had been diagnosed with an untreatable, fatal disease, her body was completely free of any evidence of the scleroderma. It was not only in remission, it had reversed. She returned home to Huntsville daring to believe she was cured.

Two years later, in the spring of 1984, she got a telephone call from a man in Athens, Alabama, saying he had scleroderma. His name was Doyle Banta and he said he taught in the local college, that he also had an insurance business and was a preacher, and that he was just about at the end of the line with his disease. Katherine had told a lot of people about what Dr. Brown had done for her, and she was delighted to be able to pass along her blessing.

Banta's scleroderma had started in a different way from Katherine's, but it had followed in the same virulent early course. He had been getting ready for bed one evening when he happened to notice what looked like a scar, about the size of a dime, on the inside of his left leg just above the ankle. As far as he could recall he had never had an injury there, and he began to wonder what it was. It happened that he was seeing a doctor at the time for a thyroid problem, and he mentioned it at his next visit. The doctor was an endocrinologist and he said he had no idea what it was, but suggested Doyle put a little Vaseline on it and see if it went away.

Instead, the scar or whatever it was got worse. By the time it reached the size of a quarter, it began to darken, and Doyle decided to take it to a dermatologist. This time the doctor diagnosed him the minute he walked into his office.

Banta had never heard of scleroderma, and at first he was relieved. "I was afraid it was skin cancer," he said.

The doctor just shook his head. "By the time this is over, you'll wish it had been—although this will hurt you just about as much as cancer." He told him the disease could drag on practically forever, but this case appeared to be moving faster than most. There was nothing that could be done for it, and he didn't even schedule another appointment. He said some doctors confirmed the diagnosis with a biopsy, but in this case he was sure that cutting into it would just make the scleroderma move all the faster. Because of that and his age, which was sixty-four, he doubted Banta would live more than another three to five years. "I wish you luck. If you find anybody that can do anything to help you, I'd sure like you to let me know."

Doyle was a naturally gregarious person, and over the course of the following months, he began hearing the names of others who suffered from the same disease. Every time he did, he made an effort to get in touch with the patient, to share stories, and to compare notes on any treatments the others might have heard about or even might have tried. The doctor's request had impressed him, and he certainly intended to let him know if he found out anything at all that might represent hope for himself or others. He also reasoned that if God helped any one of them, it was His plan that they share it with others, and Doyle meant to honor that plan.

Three-and-a-half years later, when he called Katherine Loftis, Doyle Banta became the means by which those others would learn of antibiotic therapy and Dr. Thomas McPherson Brown. It was just in the nick of time for a lot of them, including Doyle. By then his legs were the texture and color of shoe leather all the way up to the hips, and the only feeling from the mid-thigh to the toes was the agonizing sensation that the constrictive skin was about to crack and burst. Even when he went to bed, he would have to get up every couple of hours to walk and start the blood circulating again, so it was impossible to sleep through the night. At that rate, he figured the doctor's estimate was right and he didn't have more than another few months to go.

On top of the scleroderma, he had developed rheumatoid arthritis, and sometimes the pain from his joints was as savage as the agony in his skin. A family doctor put him on prednisone for the arthritis, but the circulation problem got so bad Doyle began to worry about losing both legs to gangrene. In a way, it would almost be a blessing.

He heard about Katherine Loftis because he was doing a favor for a friend, a merchant in Huntsville. Doyle had dragged himself to the friend's store to give him some advice on his expansion plans, and while they were talking, entirely by chance a man walked in who had been at college with Doyle in Abilene, Texas, some forty-four years earlier. When the classmate heard about the scleroderma, he told Doyle he knew a lady who had the same disease and had got over it.

Three weeks later, thanks to the intercession of his family doctor who pled a persuasive case on his behalf with Dr. Brown, Doyle Banta was admitted as a patient in the National Hospital in Virginia, an IV drip rack at his bedside, being given back his life. A lot of his new friends would follow him.

When I embarked on writing *The Road Back* with Tom Brown in 1988, we decided to include scleroderma in that book for the same reasons I am writing this one: the information will be useful to a lot of people who might not hear it elsewhere and who otherwise might die; and scleroderma offers a model for the connective tissue disease process in general, often responding even more dramatically than rheumatoid arthritis to antibiotic therapy. By then Tom had treated about forty patients, and he told me that every one of them had gotten better.

"In the case of scleroderma, any improvement at all is dramatic," he said, "but these improvements are truly remarkable. The patients have increased their ability to swallow. The skin on their face and hands has started to loosen up and become supple again. Those who have been caught early don't have any further progression of the disease, and those who started late have begun to reverse their condition. The most striking result has been the reversal of widespread sclerodermatous pulmonary lesions."

For Doyle Banta, by then the reversal included a steady retreat of the cracked, leathery skin to nearly the same tone as when his disease was first diagnosed. He had his old energy back, he looked ten years younger than he did just three years before, the rest of his skin was healthy again, and even the rheumatoid arthritis had left without a trace. In addition, he told me, laughing with astonishment, "Everyone I ever sent to Dr. Brown is still alive. Not one of the lupus or scleroderma patients has died, and it doesn't look like anyone is going to, at least not from those diseases. It's unbelievable to me how many people I've met who were at the brink of death, and he's brought them back to a good life."

## CHAPTER SIX

# Dr. Brown's Therapy

The family practitioner who finally diagnosed Pat Ganger's scleroderma told her they had several options in approaching a course of treatment. One would be for him to educate himself in the various therapies then in vogue, which wouldn't take that much effort as there was virtually nothing, and he would continue in his role as coordinator and primary provider of care. Another, which he said he preferred, was that she find a rheumatologist familiar with the disease who was willing to take her on as a patient.

Although Pat trusted and liked the family practitioner, after some deliberation she decided that his recommendation made sense. She went back to the popular rheumatologist who referred her to the Cleveland Clinic for a second opinion, and when that doctor agreed with the first one, the rheumatologist started her on penicillamine. In the course of searching for a diagnosis, she had been placed successively or concurrently on diuretics, Motrin, prednisone, Feldene, and a variety of other anti-inflammatories, all with no detectable effect.

By then the skin on her arms all the way up to the elbows was as hard as a Formica table top. She had a lot of trouble going up and down stairs, getting out of bed, or rising from a deep chair and sofa. Her knuckles were very sore, and soon the soreness turned into ulcers. She was fatigued even before she got out of bed in the morning. The only way she could explain it to people who had never experienced it was that it was like having a rope around her waist, and at the other end was a dead horse; everywhere she went, she had to drag the horse with her. She had no motivation to do anything, or even to think about doing anything.

When Pat began the penicillamine, she also began to hope, briefly, that the dead horse was being untethered. She found she had a little more energy, and the pain seemed somewhat milder and less persistent. She even noticed a very slight softening of the skin. But the effects lasted no more than six months before she found herself slipping back into the same condition as when she started, and then beyond that condition as she steadily worsened.

That fall, with the return of cold weather, she had her first encounter with Raynaud's syndrome. When she showed her wax-white hands and arms to the rheumatologist, he reassured her that it was a normal part of the disease, although in more typical cases it would be among the first symptoms rather than appearing as hers did in the start of the second year. It is common practice for a physician to prescribe vasodilators to relieve the painful symptoms of Raynaud's by widening the lumen of the affected blood vessels. Pat didn't know that, and for some reason the rheumatologist never suggested it to her. Maybe it was because by then the effects of the penicillamine were already beginning to fade, and he was becoming discouraged with symptomatic treatments.

It wasn't just that she was reverting to her earlier condition; once the drug stopped working, there was more tightness of the skin and greater loss in her range of motion than she had felt prior to the start of penicillamine. She was bothered more frequently with reflux, a flowing back or partial regurgitation of gastric acid, and she found it steadily more difficult to swallow food, water, even saliva. Her appearance began to change as well. One day when she and Bill were looking through an envelope of new photographs from a family get-together, she lingered in puzzlement over an alien face among the familiar ones, a woman with the pinched mouth and a strange drawing of the skin about the eyes, until she realized with a shock that she was looking at herself and seeing a stranger.

By the start of that second year, it was apparent that her disease was moving so quickly, she was going to have to face the probability of becoming incapacitated. It was a time for some serious soul-searching.

Pat knew that Bill was very uncomfortable around sick people; he didn't like visiting in hospitals and he had a hard time with funerals. She wondered how those problems would show themselves in the near future, when he would have to deal with her as an invalid, and eventually as someone who was dying.

She wondered as well how it would affect her relationship with their two children. She knew they loved her, but she kept coming back to an imagined conversation in which they would say to their spouses, "We've got to visit Mom. I promise we'll be out of there in no more than twenty minutes." She didn't want to live that way, and she dreaded the time when it would be forced upon her.

She began looking for God's purpose in what was happening to her. Their children were almost grown, the business was starting to take off, she and Bill had just bought a summer cottage on Pelee Island. Being sick was simply not on her agenda. And although she thought about it less often and still as an abstraction, neither was dying.

Up to that point in her life, her relationship with God had been fairly abstract as well. She was a believer, but her prayers were similar to messages on an answering machine, left with the expectation they would be heard, but with no dialogue and little certainty of a meaningful response. One day, she was standing at the kitchen slider and staring out across the pond behind their home, the ubiquitous question just nudging the edge of her consciousness, when God answered her call on the first ring. "Why *not* you?" She heard the words in her mind as clearly as though they had been spoken beside her.

Sitting down quickly at the table, she pondered the enigma. Try as she might to think of an answer, there was no reason she should be as blessed as she had been but remain exempt from life's vicissitudes, including pain, powerlessness, even death.

That sudden new acceptance of her burden didn't mean she was above trying to strike a bargain. After pondering her situation for a long time, she said to God, "Okay, if there's some plan in this, then I'll go along with it—providing you show me how to make an opportunity out of it."

God took her up on the offer, and in ways she never imagined.

The first such opportunity to come along was the chance to start a support group, the first of its kind in

Columbus. Up to that point, in her five years with scleroderma she had talked with just one other person who had the same disease, and that was by telephone. She knew there had to be others because, despite its relative rarity, logic told her that a city the size of Columbus would have a proportional share of the hundreds of thousands of people suffering from the same affliction.

It turned out that a local woman who ran a lupus support group through the Arthritis Foundation sent out a mailing to people who had scleroderma asking if they'd be interested in forming a similar organization. The letter may have been a result of Pat having contacted the Arthritis Foundation about a year earlier in an attempt to find just such a group; she called the woman as soon as she got her copy. Her name was Betty, and she said the reason they hadn't done this for scleroderma earlier was because they hadn't located anyone who was willing to run it. Pat volunteered on the spot; they placed an announcement in the newspaper, and twenty-nine people showed up at the very first meeting.

Pat ran the group for the next five years, and it grew to more than three times its original number. From March through October they met once a month in a conference room which Betty negotiated from one of the local health insurance companies. The reason they took off November through February was because their disease made them all particularly vulnerable to the cold, and they didn't want the meetings to become a source of discomfort or pain.

As head of the group, Pat was responsible for organizing speakers and programs. It didn't take long before they ran out of rheumatologists who could tell them anything they hadn't already heard, so more and more frequently the presentation at their meeting was whatever Pat had been able to learn about current research in their disease. There was nothing at all in the public libraries, and the only information she could find, with the help of Bill, was from local medical libraries.

In addition, Pat collected as much literature as was available from the three national scleroderma support organizations, and although it tended to be generally depressing, she shared that with the membership as well. The messages in such material seemed to divide between how badly the disease had been slighted in the past, and how exciting things were now that the situation had changed. One organization's newsletter devoted the lead article in three successive issues to the kind of professional help scleroderma patients needed most—not from their physicians, but from the attorneys in charge of planning for the disposition of their estates.

In February of 1988, she went to her rheumatologist for the usual tests by which he monitored her for any adverse reaction to the penicillamine. The urine analysis was no problem, but the blood tests were becoming progressively more painful. As the skin thickened and the vessels became more constricted, the larger veins had become too shrunken to be easy targets while the smaller surface veins, although still visually accessible, tended to collapse with the introduction of the vacuum tube. This time, despite repeated attempts, the technician was unable to get a needle through the leathery skin and into a blood supply. After a brief consultation with the doctor, she told Pat that from then on they would have to draw blood by making a small incision on the groin.

It was clear enough that the new procedure wasn't something that would be done just this one time; the monitoring took place on a monthly basis, and considering the condition of her skin, she reasoned that the incision from this month's test would hardly have time to heal before it was time to open it up again for the next one. She flatly refused. The nurse was taken aback, protesting, "But you have to." Pat answered, "You have to, but I don't. I'm stopping the treatment."

She wasn't just acting on impulse. The drug clearly was no longer working, and she felt worse with each passing day. If penicillamine was so dangerous that they had to take progressively more draconian measures just to make sure it wasn't killing her, then the ratio of risk to benefit was hopelessly out of balance. Once she got home, she walked straight to the bathroom, unscrewed the cap on the bottle of penicillamine, and dumped the remaining tablets into the toilet.

For the following ten months, she was on no medication at all. Then in early November she got a telephone call from one of the women in her group who had just read a book by a rheumatologist at the National Hospital for Orthopedics and Rehabilitation near Washington, D.C. Although *The Road Back* was about antibiotic therapy for rheumatoid arthritis, a treatment which at the time was still considered to be seriously heretical, it also contained a short chapter with two case histories about scleroderma. Pat got a copy for herself and read it through in one sitting. It made more sense to her than anything else she had

seen or heard about her disease. Bill skimmed quickly through the book the following day, and when he
finished his only comment was a question, "When are
we going?"

They discussed the treatment in the book with a
friend, a neighbor from their summer home on Pelee
Island who also had scleroderma, and he agreed to
make the pilgrimage to Washington with them. Dr.
Brown's appointment secretary at the Arthritis Clinic
of Northern Virginia told Pat that the nearest available dates were two months away, which seemed forever. But the time seemed to pass more quickly with
the hope of a positive outcome, and the trio arrived
at the National Hospital on January 2, 1989, the
Monday morning after the New Year's weekend.

There is no more rigorous test than the frigid tem-
peratures of midwinter to aggravate the symptoms of
a disease like scleroderma. Pat's Raynaud's syndrome
was at its painful worst, with her fingers turning
chalky-white and then a cyanotic blue in response to
the cold as she made her way across the hospital parking lot. The skin tightness throughout her whole
body was worse than at any time she could remember,
the fingers of both hands were curled substantially,
and the ugly crimson ulcers on her knuckles, which
had never healed in six years, were the source of
agony for fifteen or twenty minutes after even the
lightest touch.

Pat and Bill and their friend got off the elevator at
the Clinic, which was in a building immediately adja-
cent to the hospital. The receptionist logged in the
two new patients, then walked them across from her
desk to the waiting room, which was at the head of a
hallway leading down to the medical offices. Pat delib-

erately chose a seat near a window, in order for her hands to absorb whatever warmth was to be found in the ray of weak midwinter sunshine that fell across the chair.

She was barely settled in when across from the reception desk the door to the elevator opened again. This time the passengers were a small, elderly man in a wheelchair, and two very attentive women whom Pat guessed from their white uniforms were members of the clinic staff. They carefully backed the chair into the hallway, then one of them placed a cane in the old man's hand and they both helped him slowly to his feet. As he made his gingerly but deliberate way toward one of the offices about halfway down the hall, a woman seated next to Pat whispered to her in obvious reverence, "Dr. Brown."

Pat knew from the picture on the jacket of his book that Brown was no longer young, but she had hardly expected him to be so infirm. She also knew that although he still saw some of his old patients, more and more of his case load, including almost all of the new arrivals, were being handled by an associate. That one brief, disconcerting glimpse of the figure in the hallway was as close as she ever came to meeting the man who would save her life.

The treatment began on Monday morning with a brief physical examination by Dr. Cap Oliver, a longtime associate of Brown's who frequently covered for him in the final months of his life. Following the exam, Pat was hooked up for her initial session in a projected five-day regimen of intravenous antibiotic therapy. Along with the friend from Pelee Island and several other patients, most of them women with various inflammatory forms of arthritis, she sat in a small room just across the hall from the closed door of Dr. Brown's office.

They passed the time reading magazines or chatting, and some of the veterans of this therapy spoke enthusiastically to the newcomers about the progress they had made against their diseases. Pat listened with interest and even hope, but as she sat in the armchair and felt the new medicine suffusing slowly through her body, she pondered by how fragile a thread that hope was bound, and she guarded against letting it run away with her.

Seven hours later, as she was preparing to go to bed in her room at the hotel near the National Hospital, she noticed something in her legs, a change so subtle and so completely unexpected that for a moment she doubted her senses. It was a sensation which started just below her calves and extended to the feet. Incredibly, on the very first day of her treatment, the tightening of the skin around her ankles seemed to be subsiding.

During the years in which her symptoms had steadily advanced, Pat developed a series of tricks for accommodating the narrowing limits to the flexibility and agility of her body. One of them was in how she took off her shoes and socks. Because it was terribly uncomfortable to bend down, she had learned to kick off the shoes with her feet, then remove the sock from one foot by stepping on it with the heel of the other and slowly drawing up the leg. As she went through the same exercise on that first evening after the IVs, however, she realized that the ankle skin was not as tight as it had been that morning. She had grown accustomed to the feeling that her lower legs were swaddled in adhesive tape, and now she had the sense that the tape had started to unwrap.

A moment later, as she continued to undress, she realized that the ache in her wrists, which had been with her continuously for most of the past five years, was no longer there. She sat down on the edge of her bed to ponder what seemed to be happening.

Certainly there had been times in the past when the symptoms of her scleroderma had seemed better or worse, when her skin was tighter or looser, when there were small changes in her aching joints. She had been suffering from a fatal disease for six years, and the only thing different about the past two months was that she had been looking forward to a specific treatment that promised some degree of hope. Now that the therapy had started, was she so desperate for encouragement that she was reacting to nothing more than her expectations? She lay back on the bed to think about it, and in a moment she was fast asleep.

The next morning, she returned to the clinic and the therapy resumed. For the first two days she received 300 mg of clindamycin, a semisynthetic antibacterial drug used especially against gram-positive organisms. The dosage was doubled to 600 on the third day, and would be raised again to 900 for the final two. That Wednesday, after completing the third treatment in the morning, she and Bill drove across the bridge into Washington and spent the rest of the day touring every museum in the Smithsonian Institution. They saw The Spirit of St. Louis and the moon landers at Air and Space, the original Star Spangled Banner at American History, and John Smithson's tomb at the Castle. They pushed their frosty breaths ahead of them as they crossed the Mall below the Capitol to view the dinosaurs and the Hope

Diamond at the National Museum of Natural History. She hadn't had a day like that in half a decade.

Despite the fact that it was the middle of winter and Pat was on her feet for five straight hours, instead of collapsing in a heap at the end of their trek, she spent another half-hour walking around Union Station while they waited for rush-hour traffic to subside before hazarding the trip back to Virginia. When they finally returned to their hotel room, Pat looked at Bill in amazement. "This is more than wishful thinking," she said. "Two days ago, or even two years ago, I couldn't have done half of what we did this afternoon—and I'm not even tired."

The next day, halfway through the morning's therapy, Pat ran into a major pothole on her personal road back; she happened to glance down to where the IV entered her arm, and noticed it suddenly had become swollen and inflamed. The nurse saw it at the same time and told her the vein through which she was receiving the clindamycin had just closed down, or "blown," and the needle had to be withdrawn. The nurse examined her arm again the following day, and Pat was told that because of her disease, her vascular system was too fragile to finish the intravenous portion of the antibiotic therapy.

She was disappointed to not see it through the full course, but by then the evidence of significant improvements in her disease activity had long passed subtle and was overwhelming. The increase in her energy level, demonstrated so dramatically at the Smithsonian the day before, was accompanied by a corresponding retreat of the miasma of depression and hopelessness that had accumulated steadily since the onset of her disease. From the first day, she experienced none of the usual soreness from the tightened skin or from the contractures in the tendons of her hands. By the fourth day, the ulcers on her fingers had begun to heal, the first evidence visible to others that a process which had gone in only one direction for the past six years had finally changed its course.

On the afternoon of the day her IV blew, she and Bill walked across the parking lot from the clinic to enter a rear door of the National Hospital. Inside, after negotiating a series of hallways, elevator rides, and a gymnasium-like rehabilitation room full of patients and therapists, they passed through double doors into the small lobby of the Arthritis Institute, the research facility headed by Dr. Brown since his retirement as dean of medicine at George Washington University. They had come to volunteer their services in whatever way would be helpful to advance the Institute's work.

After a couple of false starts, first into a cramped laboratory where two women perched on wooden stools appeared to be conducting some kind of tests with pipettes and racks of glass vials, and then into a room which was empty except for a large, abandoned-looking electron microscope, they finally found their way to an office with a young woman who asked if she could be of help.

"That's our line," Pat said, smiling and extending her hand. "We've come over to see if *we* can help *you*."

## CHAPTER SEVEN

# Pat Ganger's Road Back

Dr. Oliver met with Pat on Friday to review the laboratory analysis of the blood taken the previous Monday morning, and to see how she had progressed on the IV therapy during the week. He told her not to be discouraged about the problem with her veins the day before, that vascular collapse was not unusual for people suffering from connective tissue disease, especially scleroderma, and he wrote her a six-month prescription for oral tetracycline in the form of pills to be taken three times a week. He also told her to continue the IV once she got home and her veins had settled down again. The latter direction was more easily said than done; back in Ohio, she could get the oral medication simply by presenting the prescription at the drug store, but even with a second prescription for IVs, she had trouble finding anyone who was willing or equipped to do them.

One day a woman came into the print shop to have some copies made, and Bill noticed that the subject of her paperwork was antibiotics. He started a conversation with her and learned she was a sales representative for a pharmaceutical firm, and that before that she had been with Caremark, a national healthcare provider licensed to perform home IVs in all fifty states. One phone call later, Pat was on her way to her second course of intravenous clindamycin therapy—but not at her house. Twice a month, the Caremark nurse came into the print shop and hooked Pat up to the IV drip rack, and for forty-five minutes she would sit in the back of the workroom, doing paperwork with her free hand, sometimes eating a sandwich or sipping a soft drink, while the medication dripped slowly into her bloodstream. If a customer or supplier happened into that part of the shop during the treatment, Bill would usually respond to their startled expressions with the explanation, "Naturally, we only let her do this on her lunch hour."

Pat had the same Caremark nurse for three years. At first there was very little conversation between them except for the amenities, a situation Pat attributed to the nurse's subdued personality. After the third or fourth treatment, that all changed. It turned out Pat was just one of several scleroderma patients the nurse had cared for over the years, although she was the first to be taking intravenous antibiotics for her disease. Like the others, Pat's skin was so hard it was a major challenge to push in the needle, and her veins were almost impossible to find except by intuition. Eventually, however, it was obvious to the nurse that Pat's case was different from the others in two important ways. First, her skin was becoming dramatically thinner and more supple, so much so that the nurse could even pinch it and manipulate it in ways that helped her find the veins by sight, and the needles entered far more freely. And second, unlike every one of the other scleroderma patients she had treated with conventional therapies, Pat was still alive.

The nurse began to bring in coworkers to meet this phenomenon and to marvel at her improvement.

Pat and Bill returned to Virginia for a follow-up visit to Dr. Oliver in the early spring. They scheduled the trip to allow themselves a couple of days at the Arthritis Institute, working with the staff and volunteers they had met in January, and this time defining specific projects on which they could be useful when they returned to Ohio. They spent time with Dr. Millicent Coker-Vann, the gracious, knowledgeable, African-born bacteriologist who ran the Institute's laboratory, and learned about her work with the mycoplasmas implicated in various forms of inflammatory arthritis and other connective tissue diseases. In a back room they worked with other volunteers on mailing lists for the Institute newsletter and helped sort through the inquiries still streaming in to Dr. Brown, more than five thousand all told, which had been generated by publication of *The Road Back* the year before.

A few days after her return from that second visit, Pat received a telephone call from Billie Eliot, the energetic, often feisty arthritis patient who ran the Institute's volunteer services. The printing shop had recently shipped her some envelopes and letterhead, and at first Pat thought that was the reason for the call. But it wasn't. Billie wanted Pat and the other volunteers to know that Dr. Brown had gone to the National Hospital for one final visit a few days earlier, this time as a patient with the bone marrow cancer he had fought for the past several years, and he had just died. Pat thought back to the frail, resolute figure she had seen in the clinic hallway not five months before, and felt a sudden, totally unexpected pang of separation. She had never met her rescuer, but Tom Brown saved her life as surely as if he had pulled her from a burning building.

It was clear from Billie's voice that she felt the same emotion far more sharply. Not only had she lost a treasured friend and mentor, but every one of Tom Brown's patients had lost their strongest and most courageous advocate, both for the infectious etiology of connective tissue disease and for the efficacy and safety of antibiotic therapy. Many of Dr. Brown's oldest patients, she feared, had also lost their only source of treatment. Dr. Brown had been as aware of this problem as anybody. He had continued seeing patients until a week before his death at the age of eighty-three.

During the months since Pat first became involved with the Arthritis Institute, she had continued running the support group in Ohio. Membership had grown to about ninety scleroderma patients from the greater Columbus area, but now things were changing. She noticed it even before her first trip to Washington, when she made it known to the members that she intended to look into the new therapy, but it was far more pronounced on her return. Her decision to explore options outside the establishment, and most particularly her subsequent improvement, was beginning to affect her relationship with the other members in ways she could never have anticipated. The restoration of her appearance, her mobility, her energy, and her state of mind were visible for all of the other members to see, but as much as those changes impressed the nursing professionals, they seemed to have far less impact on her fellow patients—or, perhaps more to the point, on the doctors who were treating them. The situation became so strained that Pat had trouble finding physicians who even would come to speak at their monthly meetings. She suspected it was because they knew she was on an unconventional therapy and, more offensive yet, that she obviously was getting better.

She sensed that the other members were becoming remote. The condition that originally brought them together had remained unchanged for the rest of them, but Pat's recovery, instead of providing a motivational model, now seemed to be having the opposite result of driving her out of the group. Rather than trusting the evidence of their own direct observation, the others elected to continue their reliance on whatever therapy their doctors directed—in some cases, no doubt, because they could not get permission from the doctors to make a change.

The Gangers thought back on how they had learned about scleroderma in their own lives, and it was not because they had the benefit of input from Pat's own physicians or had witnessed any improvement in her peers. The specialist who gave Pat her diagnosis named a disease neither of them had ever heard of, and he provided virtually no useful information about what to expect or how to treat it. When Pat read *The Road Back*, Dr. Brown was a stranger and the two scleroderma case histories in the book, of Doyle Banta and Katherine Loftis, were about people she had never met. She had chosen to believe them— perhaps, she now thought, because the book also offered a plausible model for the mechanism of the disease as well as its treatment.

The way they had chosen to manage that part of their lives was a lot like the way they had taught themselves the printing business, by throwing themselves into the middle of it, deciding on their own what worked, and discovering the rules as they went along.

Pat persisted with the group, but after three more years of vain attempts to lead by example, she attended one last meeting. "I've told you everything about scleroderma you need to know," she said. "I've gotten better in front of you, but you still act as though you'd prefer to think of your situation as hopeless. You've chosen to rely more on what your doctors have told you than on what you've seen. There are lots of other people who do want to learn about the only therapy that works, and I'm going to start spending my time telling them about it."

One of the members agreed to take over Pat's stewardship, and the support group continues today under the aegis of the Arthritis Foundation.

By the time Pat left that organization, she and Bill were deeply involved with the Arthritis Institute, and things there didn't seem to be going much better.

There had been a precipitous decline in support since Dr. Brown's death, and unease at the loss of his leadership deteriorated to the petty territorialism that often accompanies anxiety and grief.

## CHAPTER EIGHT

# A Husband's Story

Despite the absence of any useful information from their doctor about what to expect from this strange new development in their lives, at about the time of Pat's diagnosis, Bill began to notice other disturbing changes in his wife, particularly in her attitude toward daily living. She had always had a lot of energy, but now she was slower to get out of bed in the morning and she would tire earlier and more frequently during the course of the day, even if she hadn't been doing anything to account for the fatigue. It was as though she had become disheartened by the uncertainty, and now she was just going to lie down and give in to being sick.

He decided this surrender to the disease was bad for her, that it was a form of giving up, and he made up his mind to do everything he could to help her fight it. There didn't seem to be much either of them could do about the attitude of the doctors, but Pat's own attitude was another matter. Bill knew about the connection between physical and spiritual health, and he was determined to get his wife back on her feet. The couple talked it over, and despite how poorly she felt they agreed she should return to work. It was a joint decision, but they both knew when they made it that there would be times when Bill would have to really push to keep her going.

Pat's job, as his own, was at their storefront print shop, so it wasn't as though she were going to work every day for someone else. They had started the business together, and although Bill could have carried on without her at his side, even during the worst parts of her illness they still went down there every day, because they both knew how important it was that she keep active and maintain a positive outlook. There was only one other employee, and it was in the nature of the business that all three of them had to know how to do everything. Pat didn't spare herself or expect any special treatment; she worked on the front counter, set type, took her turn making coffee, proofread, sent out bills, balanced the books, dealt with suppliers, ran the machines.

The years rolled by and her condition worsened, but still no one told them anything useful that they could do about it. At the outset, they had done what most people do when they or someone close to them develops a serious, debilitating, painful, progressive disease: they just turned it all over to the doctor who had given it a name, assuming that Pat's case was at the top of his daily list of problems to solve and things to do. After five years, Bill realized that was hardly the case, that the doctors had either written her off or they hardly thought of her at all. If Pat were to go anywhere but continually downhill, it was going to be up to someone else to change the direction her disease had clearly taken. The obvious problem was that there *was* no one else—besides, of course, himself.

In 1987, he set out on his own to learn whatever he could about the disease that was changing his wife's

appearance and threatening to take her away entirely. His commitment tapped a resource of resolve that
surprised even him, and although the quest began
almost casually, in a few months he found himself systematically working his way through the stacks in the
medical library at Ohio State University. Most of what
he found was way over his head, but he figured they
would both get smarter as he went along, so he read
whatever he could find and brought home the most
interesting stuff for Pat. It wasn't much at first—some
definitions, a few case histories—but then he began to
branch out into books about connective tissue,
rheumatology, dermatology, blood testing, whatever
areas were related to the disease.

Pat wasn't too enthusiastic about Bill's project when
it began, mostly because in addition to being sick she
felt confused and overwhelmed. After all, if scleroderma had stumped the specialists who had spent
their lives in the study of medicine, what chance did
a couple of amateurs have to uncover anything that
could possibly make a difference?

In addition to that form of discouragement, they
both had to constantly battle her lethargy from the disease itself. Bill took over most of the responsibilities at
home, including shopping, cleaning, preparing meals,
and looking after the needs of the children. Despite
the way she felt and the improbability that anything
either of them did or learned would make a bit of difference to the outcome, she gradually began to take
more interest in the information her husband was
bringing home from the library. She realized as he did
that even if the exercise proved ultimately futile, for
the present it gave them both a sense that they
remained somehow in charge of what was happening

in their lives, that they weren't entirely out of control if they could still keep their hands on the wheel.

Throughout this whole process, and in the face of everything they learned, Bill remained an extreme optimist. In looking back, part of the reason may have been that he was in complete denial about her prognosis from the outset. Neither one of them really understood just how serious scleroderma was until they found out for themselves, and by then he had somehow developed a strong, sometimes even ferocious, sense that they could make a difference after all. Perhaps it was true that in the land of the blind, the one-eyed man is king. More than that, he felt empowered by the process of self-education, the first step toward taking charge of the disease that had changed their lives.

When her energy started coming back to her, Pat found that she and Bill just worked all the harder. They would get up at seven o'clock every day, and go to sleep at one-thirty or two o'clock the following morning, and sometimes the only things they had a chance to talk about during the entire day were the business and her disease. Their commitments to understanding scleroderma, to beating it, and then to helping others were consuming and insatiable. By now their children were grown and pretty much on their own, so the demands on Pat as mother and homemaker were fewer than at the time of onset. Then there was the fact that Dr. Brown was dying. He had given her the only real help for her disease that she had ever received, and when it became obvious that his voice was about to be silenced, both she and Bill sometimes felt nearly desperate in their urgency to help spread the story.

Pat had heard about Dr. Brown and started taking the treatment in 1989. She got immediate results, followed by months of more gradual improvement, but if Bill thought the change in her health meant that he would get back his wife of years before, he had underestimated how far-reaching the impact of her disease had been for both of them. Even though she was getting better, he came to realize they had both embarked on a journey, and neither of them would ever return to where it had begun.

## CHAPTER NINE
# What Return Can We Make?

---

In the spring of 1990, a year after Tom Brown's death, Pat Ganger helped organize a meeting in Chicago of about a dozen physicians from around the country who were practicing his antibiotic protocol, principally for rheumatoid arthritis. Sponsored by the Arthritis Institute, the conference provided the doctors with a forum for trading insights gained from their clinical experience and for discussing the future of the therapy. By that time, *The Road Back* had been out for two years and the doctors who had contacted the Arthritis Institute to inquire about the protocol or to say they were offering the treatment numbered in the hundreds. But the politics were still so intense that only a relative handful of physicians had dared to go public with their apostasy, and even fewer were willing to take time off from their practices and pay their own way to the middle of the country for a meeting with their peers.

Among those who did attend were two osteopaths, Joe Mercola from nearby Schaumburg, Illinois, and John Sinnott from Ida Grove, Iowa. Dr. Mercola had several dozen rheumatoid arthritis patients and Dr. Sinnott, who worked for a time in Arlington with Dr. Brown, had subsequently treated somewhere around three hundred patients. Pat was impressed by their accessibility and open enthusiasm for the therapy. She also calculated that the trip from Columbus to Chicago had taken her only half the time of her numerous journeys to Washington, and with the decline of the Arthritis Institute following Dr. Brown's death, her other incentive for the long trek east had begun to diminish as well. It was still too early to give up on the Arthritis Institute, but by the end of the conference she was greatly relieved to know that there were alternatives for the same treatment if she should ever need them.

During the course of her work with the Arthritis Institute, Pat had come to know the names of other volunteers scattered around the country who were doing the most to keep the organization alive, and they stayed in frequent contact with each other by telephone. A few months after the Chicago conference, she had the idea that key members of this cadre should try to schedule their next visit to Arlington at the same time so they could meet in person and get to know each other better. But when she called the Arthritis Clinic to see what she could organize, Dottie told her that unless they wanted to wait for several months, the earliest available dates were in December, not a popular time of year for patients with cold sensitivity to leave the shelter of their homes. Just before Christmas, Pat wound up at the National Hospital with only one other out-of-towner, an arthritis/polymyositis patient from St. Louis, Missouri, named Ethel Snooks.

As usual, Pat and Bill scheduled their trip so that they could spend the weekend working at the Arthritis Institute, as did Ethel and her husband Ray.

By Sunday night, the two couples returned to their motel, exchanged weary goodnights, and headed for their separate rooms. But when Pat and Bill were alone and able to share their feelings, they quickly agreed they felt as though they had spent the past two days doing work that should have been completed in twenty minutes, and they sensed that Ray and Ethel were equally frustrated by the politics and indecisiveness that followed the loss of Tom Brown's leadership. Together they walked down the hall and knocked on the Snookses' door.

Ray and Ethel had already gotten ready for bed, but they invited the Gangers in and the two couples shared their concerns for the future. They both had solid, pragmatic reasons for their anxiety that went far beyond the questions of who was in charge of their volunteer efforts or the warring personalities within the Institute. Pat and Ethel had no doubts that Tom Brown's therapy had saved their lives, along with the lives of thousands of others who had either been his patients or whose physicians had treated them with his protocol. At that point, the organization Tom Brown had left behind was the only such group in America, or, indeed the entire world, dedicated to the concept that their respective diseases were infectious or that they could be treated safely and effectively with antibiotic therapy. If the Institute were allowed to fail, they both feared that Tom Brown's theory and treatment would die as well, and they and the millions of others suffering from rheumatoid arthritis, lupus, scleroderma, and other connective tissue diseases would be bereft of either advocacy or recourse. It was already hard enough to find a doctor willing to look at the evidence or to read Dr. Brown's protocol, much less his book, and there was enormous peer pressure on those physicians who broke ranks with the establishment and actually offered the therapy to patients who requested it. The Arthritis Institute, however embattled and dispirited, was the last place on earth where the patient still had a voice, and they dreaded the prospect that it might fall into silence.

The Gangers and the Snookses talked late into the night, but by the time they parted the way still was far from clear. The only course they could agree on was to be patient, to continue serving their common cause in the ways they were permitted by the institute's leadership, to search for other avenues of service, and, most of all, to pray. They did all of those things, still serving the Arthritis Institute during their trips to Arlington, over the course of the next two years.

The problems there continued to worsen, and by the spring of 1992, in consultation with other active volunteers from around the United States and Canada who shared the same concerns, Pat and Ethel took the first step towards a new course of action. A dozen patients and supporters of Dr. Brown's therapy met at the Snookses' house just outside St. Louis with the purpose of planning a specific program in support of their cause. Before any program was actually begun, each participant agreed to write everyone else they knew with a connective tissue disease and enlist their opinion on whether to proceed. Some four hundred letters were mailed, and one-quarter of the addressees replied; the consensus was overwhelmingly in favor of moving ahead. A second meeting was held in October, this time at the Gangers' in Ohio, and The Road Back Foundation was incorporated in that state, with Pat as president, the following January.

Initial financial support came primarily from the hundred-odd patients who had responded to the letter, even though it contained no solicitation or even mention of money. Later in the year, when an update to *The Road Back* was published by Brown's co-author as *The Arthritis Breakthrough*, the new volume contained a brief description of the Foundation's work, and the public contributions increased.

The Foundation's stated purpose was to serve as an information resource for people who would have a hard time learning about their legitimate therapeutic options from any other source. Pat and Ethel recognized that Dr. Brown was still anathema in the rheumatology community, and rather than exacerbate existing rancorous divisions by turning his name into a banner, they deliberately set about to prove his case by other means. They combed the respected, mainstream, peer-reviewed medical literature for every study they could find in support of antibiotic therapy, the role of mycoplasmas, or an infectious etiology for connective tissue disease.

Even in the short time since Dr. Brown's death, the body of such data had grown substantially. Breedveld's paper on the Netherlands study had appeared in *The Journal of Rheumatology* in 1990, triggering a quick succession of other study proposals and editorials on a possible infectious etiology for the disease and the future role of antibiotics. By the time The Road Back Foundation was getting organized just two years later, an editorial appeared in that same respected publication under the title, "The Microbial Cause of Rheumatoid Arthritis: Time to Dump Koch's Postulates," referring to the traditional steps for establishing a micro-organism as the cause of a disease.

Koch's postulates required that the same cause be found in all cases; that it be isolable from the host and grown in pure culture; that it reproduce the original disease when introduced into a susceptible host; and that it be found in the host afterward. Part of that sounds like what Albert Sabin did with his two laboratory mice way back in 1939, but of course the problem then was reproducibility. More than half a century later, the authors of the editorial (Drs. Paul L. J. Tan and Margot A. Skinner of the University of Auckland School of Medicine) asked whether this were a legitimate test or even possible in a disease as complex, selective, and elusive as rheumatoid arthritis.

The Road Back Foundation began publishing its quarterly newsletter, focusing less on the role of Dr. Brown as a pioneer and heretic, and more on the case for and against the infectious theory and antibiotic therapy in the current literature. Pat found that the positive evidence far outweighed the negative and, even more significantly, that it was continuing to accumulate at a steadily increasing rate.

The new organization grew in pretty much the same way, with one patient telling another, word passing from family to family, doctor to doctor. It was a slow process, but because Pat and Ethel were careful not to overextend the support base, it was also a manageable one; they were reasonable in setting the goals for their new organization and methodical in meeting them. From the day that it began, the Foundation never operated in the red.

The first year was especially difficult because everyone was getting used to working together in a new context, and, unlike the effort directed by Dr. Brown, this movement was driven entirely by the patients.

The task was made bearable by their knowledge that the best was yet to come. The seeds Tom Brown had sown were now rooted elsewhere as well, not just among his loyal patients but in Congress and among medical researchers who could no longer ignore his life's work.

In the same month The Road Back Foundation came into official existence in Ohio, a report was issued in Washington on "Mycoplasma Research, Infectious Disease Theory Research, or Antibiotic Clinical Trials," over the signature of Bernadine Healy, M.D., soon-to-retire director of the National Institutes of Health (NIH). The report answered a request from the Senate Committee on Appropriations from a decade earlier for a detailed accounting of NIH research into mycoplasma-related causes of rheumatoid arthritis. The prologue recalled that during 1983, the NIH "actively worked with Dr. Thomas McPherson Brown, Dr. Howard Clarke, and their colleagues at the Arthritis Institute of the National Hospital in Arlington, Virginia, who were applying for research grant support for a clinical trial to assess the efficacy of tetracycline treatment of rheumatoid arthritis. They were unsuccessful in obtaining grant support."

The affable, downright collegial description of that process might lead a naive or casual reader to believe the NIH shared in Tom Brown's disappointment, but that conclusion would be as inaccurate as the report writer's recollection of his associate's name (Dr. Harold Clark.) In fact, the NIH's own peer review committee visited the Institute, inspected the facility, talked at length with Brown and Clark about the rationale and design of their proposed study, and returned to Bethesda with a recommendation that it be funded. The recommendation was ignored, and Tom Brown would never learn that it was the NIH administration, and not his colleagues, who had deprived him of this final chance to prove his case within his lifetime.

(When Dr. Healy resigned her job a short time later, she complained publicly about the frustration she had experienced in attempting to manage her consortium of fiefdoms, and she warned of the consequences that were sure to result if the ducal powers of the NIH continued putting politics, power, and private gain ahead of the public interest.)

Although very little happened in the first four years covered by the NIH report, the funding for infectious arthritis research grew sixfold between 1987 and the end of the decade in question, accounting for nearly eight million dollars in grant awards in 1992 alone.

The NIH report to Congress culminated in a description of the long-awaited study of minocycline in rheumatoid arthritis (MIRA), funded at four million dollars through seven related contracts to six clinical centers and one coordinating center, a far grander version of the proposal the NIH had rejected from Tom Brown a decade earlier, and every bit as controversial before it ever started. The report ended with the forecast that the MIRA study "should answer many questions about the safety and efficacy of long-term administration of minocycline to patients with rheumatoid arthritis." The clinical work was already finished, and it was expected the results would be assembled and analyzed in time for reporting at the 1993 annual meeting of the American College of Rheumatology in San Antonio, Texas.

Pat Ganger and Ethel Snooks, along with this writer and some half-dozen other of Dr. Brown's former patients, colleagues, and members of The Road Back Foundation, wouldn't have missed that meeting for the world.

## CHAPTER TEN

# Whistle

I first heard of a patient named Cynthia Dale from Dr. Trentham in the fall of 1995. At the time he told me about her, The Road Back Foundation's scleroderma study had already begun at Harvard Medical School, but Cynthia was not a part of it. Trentham had started her on minocycline therapy three years before the study began, his first scleroderma patient on the treatment. He told me she had done "astonishingly" well and he thought her story would make a good case history for the next edition of *The Arthritis Breakthrough*, which had a short section on the disease. The idea of a book on just scleroderma had not yet occurred to either of us.

When I told Cynthia the reason for my call she was immediately responsive and we set a date to meet for lunch at the Whiton House, a restaurant in a rambling, post-colonial inn beside the old King's Highway in the coastal village of Hingham, Massachusetts, just south of Boston. I didn't know what to expect and was pleasantly relieved when she turned out to be a personable, dark-haired, well-dressed woman, probably in her mid-to-late thirties, with a good handshake, plenty of steady, straightforward eye contact, obvious intelligence—and no apparent trace of the disease.

We passed the first few minutes in small talk, looking at the menu, and assessing each other. She was an executive, I learned, with a major national retailer of upscale casual clothing. She lived nearby with her husband who freelanced in the communications field and their nine-year-old daughter. When the waitress came for our orders, Cynthia asked for a Caesar salad and I chose the eggs Benedict, just the right selections, I thought, for an attractive young professional clearly intent on staying trim, and a writer who, perhaps just as clearly, was not.

Partly because our purpose required her to do most of the talking, I finished luncheon first and reached into my briefcase for a recorder, which I placed on the table between us. I asked her permission to tape the rest of our conversation, and she agreed, but when I started the machine and asked for her name, I realized from the quizzical, nearly startled expression on her face that our interview was already in trouble.

She told me she was glad to offer her case history, but not if it included her name. It was not an altogether unexpected reaction; I had run into the same thing while gathering case histories on rheumatoid arthritis, and in all such instances but one, I had declined the interview. Without the name of a real person, the reader has no assurances the story is accurate, complete, or even true. On the other hand, patient privacy is an issue in discussing any disease, and it may be axiomatic that the more serious the subject, the less the likelihood of openness. Systemic scleroderma was untreatable, of unknown etiology, and came with the prospect of disfigurement, suffering, and death. Like a plague of the Dark Ages, the mechanism of transmission was equally unknown as its cause, and despite all the evidence to the contrary, for those friends and associates who were inclined to be fearful, it was not hard to imagine it could be caught by something as innocent as a handshake, a touch, or even the sharing of the same air.

Cynthia told me she hadn't confided her situation in anyone outside her immediate family, not even her parents. It wasn't just that she was a highly private person. Her father was struggling with prostate cancer and he had plenty of problems of his own. Besides, he had just retired and they were heading into that part of their lives where they would hope their children were physically and emotionally independent, that they were making it on their own.

As much as she didn't want to unfairly burden those she loved with more protracted anxiety or grief than they could handle, she equally wanted to protect her professional life against the unfounded fears of others, including any premature assumptions that she could no longer function effectively in her job. No one at work knew she had been diagnosed with a fatal disease, much less its name, and if any of her coworkers suspected something was the matter they had never asked her what it was. When I expressed some surprise at that last statement, she responded with a cool, level look and said quietly, "You don't know me; they do. I'm not someone you'd ask."

I put the recorder back in my briefcase and we chatted some more, but no longer with our original intention, while she finished eating. Despite feeling some disappointment at not hearing her story in detail or being able to use it in a future edition of the book on arthritis, I was glad for the opportunity to meet her and to see her in such obvious good health. She was an important figure in the sequence of events leading to the study; I was sure that her success with minocycline therapy had been a factor in David Trentham's agreement to undertake the clinical trial.

I don't now remember if Cynthia told me at that meeting whether she had read *The Road Back* or *The Arthritis Breakthrough* or indeed if she had even heard of them, but neither book had a direct connection with her starting the treatment that would save her life.

A year and a half later, the Harvard study was completed and David Trentham once again suggested I include Cynthia's story in whatever I wrote about the disease. I told him I doubted she would change her mind, but he urged me to give it another try. I called from Ohio a few days later, and this time, after I told Cynthia some of the recent background, I offered her Plan B. I said I felt her case was so important to the history of the treatment that I was willing to hide her identity in whatever I wrote. She listened quietly, and after a moment's reflection she said, "You don't need to. You can use my name."

Three days later, we met again at the Whiton House. She was as cordial as ever, and she couldn't have looked more fit. More than that, I sensed an optimism, even an excitement, about our purpose that had been missing when we met the first time. When the waitress came, Cynthia ordered the eggs Benedict, and if there was any risk that I had forgotten, she said, "That's what you had when we ate here before." Naturally, I ordered the Caesar salad.

During lunch I told her what I knew about the results of the Harvard study, but by tacit agreement we carefully stayed away from the subject of her own experience with the disease; we both realized that it was not going to be an easy story to tell, and a crowded restaurant was the wrong venue. After we ate, when I mentioned my misgivings, she immediately agreed and suggested we drive the short distance to her house. She introduced me to her husband, and when he went back to his upstairs office we sat in the living room and I again reached into my briefcase.

This time, when I turned on the recorder, the first thing she said was, "My name is Cynthia Dale."

She said she had the first symptoms of her disease in September of 1991. They were mostly joint problems. Then her hands started to swell and even when she took her rings off the pain continued almost steadily. Often she would wake up in the night and would have to get up and stand beside her bed, shaking her arms and kneading her knees because the circulation was shut off and they felt as though they had gone to sleep.

She tolerated those symptoms for four or five months before she decided they were serious enough that it would be worth seeing a doctor. Her family practitioner did a series of tests and eventually sent her to a rheumatologist who did some more tests and named the disease. The whole process took about a year. The rheumatologist then explained to her, after a fashion, what it meant.

He said she was seriously ill, and he gave her a little brochure from the hospital which told her virtually nothing. He said that scleroderma was a connective tissue disease, that there were very few people who had it, and that there was no cure. Over the course of the next several visits he gave her a series of tests—

lung tests, heart tests, stress tests—which he explained had nothing to do with helping her get better but were benchmarks so that over the course of the disease he could chart the deterioration of her organs. He said he could give her some penicillamine, but he didn't think it would do any good, and he left it at that. Beyond the gloomy hint in his explanation of the benchmarks, he told her nothing specific about what to expect, and never mentioned mortality. Apparently he was willing to let her find that part out all by herself.

As Cynthia learned more about the disease from other sources, she began to think about the possibility of dying. Although she was not particularly worried for herself, she became terrified at the possibility that she might not be there for her daughter. Because by then she didn't want to ask the rheumatologist, she went back to her general practitioner and confronted him point-blank, "Will I see my daughter graduate?" When he lowered his eyes and then his whole head and said he didn't know, that there was no way of telling, she had her answer.

The next question was, how long? She pondered her situation, then tried a new strategy, this time on the rheumatologist. At her next visit, she said, "I'm really sick, aren't I?"

"Yes, you are," he answered.

"Am I going to make it?"

He hesitated. "Well, some people make it to their seventies. There are no articles or references on this that will really help tell you."

The strongest emotion she felt after these exchanges was complete, utter frustration that there was no one who could help her, not with the disease, not with describing it fully, not even with her normal need for some general map of the future landscape. Instead of despairing, Cynthia decided almost at that moment that she had to take matters into her own hands, starting with a search for whomever she could find, wherever they might be, who could tell her something about the disease. She would have flown anywhere in the world to talk with anyone who could offer her hope or, at the very least, educate her in what was happening and what lay ahead.

She discovered the truth soon enough. From her business experience she knew how to get information, and proceeded to collect and devour everything she could get her hands on related to the disease. In the course of that search, she found a notice in the *Boston Globe* for a clinical trial on scleroderma of something called photopheresis, with an 800 number for the Scleroderma Federation in Peabody. She called, and when they heard that she was near Boston, they encouraged her to become a part of the trial. The next day she received a large package of material, but it was so technical she could understand almost none of it.

Cynthia went to see the doctor in charge of the study just once. He was a dermatologist, and he told her she was a perfect candidate. He assured her the treatment was promising and that the timing was just right, that she wasn't too far into her disease. The attempts to persuade by soothing had just the opposite of their intended effect. She felt uneasy, even put off, not least because she recalled reading somewhere that photopheresis had already been proven in previous trials to be ineffective for scleroderma. She told the doctor that she wanted to gather more information.

Ironically, the suggestion that photopheresis did not work was among the few understandable things in all the material she had gotten from the Scleroderma Federation. In looking through it again, she found an article about Dr. David Trentham at Beth Israel Hospital in Boston, which also identified him as president of the International Society for Rheumatic Therapies, and, in the second, more careful reading, it was apparent that Trentham had serious misgivings about the experimental therapy. She decided that if she were to consider the study she should talk to him first for his perspective on what it was all about. She called his office for an appointment.

The first thing Dr. Trentham said when they met was that Cynthia had "raging scleroderma," and that if she had come to him three months sooner he might have been able to give her better news. He told her there were five options, and he discussed each one of them in detail. The one they settled on was a combination approach: penicillamine, which is an amino acid used in lead poisoning, some forms of arthritis, and against the formation of stones in the urinary tract, for the possibility that it might offer some symptomatic relief; and the antibiotic minocycline. (Although she started out with them both, Trentham would drop the penicillamine, so she was on just minocycline for the final year.)

It turned out that Dr. Trentham had trained the rheumatologist who had seen her first and diagnosed her disease, and he made no secret of his dismay with the way he had handled the case. The patient's morale and state of mind are central factors in any disease process, and Trentham was appalled that the rigorous organic tests were explained by such a hopeless, fatalistic rationale. In all the years he would treat her, although he sampled her blood and urine at every visit, he never put Cynthia through a similar examination to the ones she had endured for her benchmarks; he said she'd had enough. Besides, they weren't treating her disease just to watch her fail.

By the time they began the therapy, Cynthia's scleroderma had advanced far beyond its initial symptoms. Her hands, already tight and swollen, had become so covered with red rashes and bumps that her husband said they looked like they had been dipped in boiling acid. She suffered from acute Raynaud's syndrome, had lost the fine hair on her arms and legs, and the skin on her face was as tight and smooth as if it had been through several face-lifts. Her knees were very tight and painful as well, and if she got up in the middle of the night she first had to lubricate them just so she could walk.

She had to get up often. Her daughter, then six, knew Mommy was sick and she was showing signs of anxiety, including sometimes waking in the middle of the night and calling to her. When that happened, it would take Cynthia forever to get herself out of bed, to oil the skin of her knees until they were flexible enough that she could put her feet on the floor, then to find her way painfully down the dark hall and into her daughter's room, where she would sit patiently on the edge of her bed, stroking her hair and assuring the frightened little girl that her mother was still there.

Even after she began Dr. Trentham's treatment, the tightness and painful sensitivity continued to spread and eventually it was all over her body—her back, her stomach, the rest of her legs, everywhere—and if anyone touched her, it felt as though she had been stabbed with pins.

Perhaps as a part of coping with her pain and the sense of loss that accumulated with the decline in her mobility, she felt an enormous need for privacy. The decision to not share what was happening with anyone beyond her husband and daughter proved progressively more challenging in practice; as director of retail stores for her employer she had a very visible job, and now she developed a sense of being constantly scrutinized by colleagues who had come to know her when her energy levels were much higher, before the disease slowed down her body and burdened her with so much pain, before she had difficulty picking up a pencil and needed to use two hands just to hold a drinking glass. Her life at work became a balancing act between performing the tasks which were expected of her and keeping up the pretense of normalcy while in fact the opposite was the case, and her whole life, even her body, was less and less in her control.

It occurred to her that her condition might have generated some speculation within the company, perhaps even some gossip, but no one besides her boss ever asked her if she was all right, and if there was any such talk, none of it ever got back to her.

Beyond the pain, one of the hardest parts of conducting her day-to-day business was impatience. She wanted everything to be done, to have closure, before she finally lost all control and the disease devoured her. She began obsessing on the things that wouldn't be taken care of if she died. She and her husband had a long conversation about what he had to do when the time finally came, and they started making specific plans for her death.

One result of those plans was that she started writing a series of short letters to her daughter. A little girl of six has one set of concerns and needs, and Cynthia knew a child of twelve would have others. When those times of change arrived—reaching young womanhood, starting high school, her first date, getting married—it was Cynthia's hope that her daughter could read the letter that applied to each new stage of life and hear her mother speaking to her, guiding her, still loving her. (She had tears in her eyes as she told me this part of the story, but she sat ramrod-straight on the sofa and her voice was quiet and firm, never wavering. I was beginning to know her.)

The penicillamine or the minocycline upset her stomach slightly, and she compensated by eating more. She suggested to Dr. Trentham that one of the medicines might have a side effect of making her gain weight, but he said no such side effect had been reported in the literature. She thought about it and decided that subconsciously she was eating to hide the symptoms of the disease. She didn't want anyone to see what she had, and especially she didn't want to upset her parents or to have them worry.

Throughout this process, she continually balanced what she knew and thought against how she felt. As painful as her condition was and as bleak as her prognosis, she still didn't *feel* like she was dying. She kept asking herself, "Why does everything I read or hear about my disease tell me I'm dying, when I don't feel it?" She decided that the answer was that she was in denial. She had no trouble recognizing that she had to get her life in order, that

her will had to be up-to-date, that she had responsibilities to her husband and her child to help them in
whatever way possible after she was gone. She tried
organizing all the people around her on her job to
make sure that everything would continue to go
smoothly when she was no longer able to carry on.
In every part of her life she felt that overwhelming
need for closure, for everything to be under control
and to have a predictable ending. But she still could
not come to terms with the actual process, with the
letting go, with the acceptance that she was no
longer in control.

Her boss, a woman Cynthia respected and
admired, came down to her office one day and asked,
"What's happening to you?"

After months of successfully holding the world
around her in check, she was startled by the question
and must have looked confused or even panicky.

"I've lost you," the boss went on. "You've become a
whole different person."

Unable to control herself any longer, Cynthia burst
into tears. "I'm sick," she said. "I'm trying to deal with
it, and I'm doing the best I can. Am I being bad? Is
there something that I need to do?"

It was obvious the boss was shocked, but as quickly
as Cynthia had capitulated to her feelings, she recovered and firmly drew the line. She said she would discuss the problem only as far as it was affecting her job.
Her boss assured her it wasn't affecting her job at
all—it was just that she had been acting somehow dif-
ferently than she ever had before, and the two women
had known each other for a long time. The boss never
asked about the specific nature of the problem; she
knew better than to cross over into Cynthia's person-

al space. With no place else for the conversation to go, a moment later it ended.

Now they knew something was wrong. And now Cynthia knew that they were very worried about her. She pondered the passing of this latest milestone.

One of the reasons she was unwilling to let anyone in to talk about her condition or her feelings or her future, she realized, was because she carried such an enormous burden of grief at her slow erosion and the pending ultimate loss that she never dared to relax the iron grip on her emotions.

Christmas came. Cynthia found herself nearly overwhelmed by the need for just the right words, to tell her daughter what she felt she needed to say, not just to reassure her that they could all deal with this as it happened, but even to show her precisely how, down to the smallest detail. She needed to tell her little girl where to find the strength so that she would endure, what she needed to do and think and feel so that her life would continue.

She had the same problem communicating her feelings to her husband; it was hard for her to face the certainty of his coming grief when she would no longer be there to help him through it. She told him she hoped he would get married again, and even as she said it she had the terrible feeling that she was organizing everyone right down to every possible future thought or feeling. There are some things in life, she thought to herself, that you can't just look up in the Yellow Pages, and she would become impatient or even angry at such times for what she came to think of, privately, as her operational approach to dealing with her feelings. It always came back to the same issues. She didn't want to be a burden on people. She didn't want people feeling sorry for her. She just wanted to make sure that everything and everybody were going to be okay.

Then one day, several weeks into the therapy, something different started to happen.

Cynthia didn't notice it as quickly as Dr. Trentham did, but after looking at her blood results at the end of one of her visits, he told her she was getting better. At first she thought he must be wrong, but then she realized that the pain had started to lessen. A few more weeks passed, and as they both watched her body, the message became clearer. However subtly, the ravaged skin had begun to heal. The swelling was starting to subside. The tightness slowly abated. She could hardly believe what was happening.

Cynthia grew up as a Catholic but had left the church when she got to college. She realized she had acquired new values and suddenly the unquestioned faith of her childhood stopped making sense—if it ever did. But all that began to change again when she had a child of her own, well before the onset of her illness, and she and her husband agreed on the need to give their daughter's life an anchor in religion. She recalled the feelings she had gone through at the time she had separated from Catholicism, and probably some of them were still valid, but she was already busy with her career and she didn't have the time to search for the perfect answer; she wound up going back to the Catholic church.

During her illness there had been lots of times when she would leave work and go to the church and pray. She prayed for peace and acceptance. She prayed for strength. She prayed her gratitude for the life God had given her. She prayed for her daughter, her husband, her family. She prayed for courage, for endurance, for grace, not just for herself but for them all. She prayed for others in her life who had terrible problems like her own. She prayed for strangers, people who would remain forever unknown to her, with whom she shared this terrible disease. And sometimes, although not always, she prayed that if it were God's will, she would be made well.

And it was happening.

"You get back what you put in," she told me. "That's how it works. Dr. Trentham will say it's the medication, and I say yes, it is, but Somebody's helping us do all this. The affirmation in my faith and the improvement in my health came together. Now my faith isn't going to go away and neither is my life. You've got to believe in whatever you've got to believe in."

The first real sign that her disease was reversing was that when something touched her skin, it didn't feel as though someone were stabbing it with a needle. Then the swelling started going down. The whole process took about six months, but the pain started going away within the first several weeks. Cynthia had always had a little arthritis in her knees, but soon after the initial signs of remission she found she could squat down, could kneel, and when playing with her daughter or working at home eventually could even walk on her knees around the floor.

Then her energy started to come back, and she couldn't believe that she was actually looking forward to getting out of bed in the morning. At work there is a long corridor that she had to travel frequently, and as she got sicker she had become slower and slower whenever she had to make the journey—all the time trying to look laid-back and efficient, keeping up the painful pretense that she wasn't sick at all. Some days she had even wondered if she would be able to make it to the end. When she started getting better there was a fleeting, magical moment when she realized she was actually picking up speed, that it was no longer a charade, that she was again becoming the person who, for so many painful months, she had merely pretended to be.

There were lots of such moments, and she treasured every one of them. In the depths of her illness, because of tendon contractures her fingers had curled down toward the palm like claws, and she needed to spread them apart and wrap each finger around whatever object she wanted to hold. She hadn't been able to grasp a toothbrush because her fingers couldn't close around it firmly enough, and anyway she couldn't open her mouth wide enough to get it in without forcing it. During the worst two years, she didn't go to the dentist because she couldn't tolerate sitting in a chair while he forced her mouth open.

Then one day she realized that her hands were straightening out. On her visits to Dr. Trentham, the first thing he would do was take hold of her hands and move the fingers, and every time he did it he'd get a wider range of motion, and he'd say, "Look, look!" His enthusiasm and delight reminded her of the little piggy game that parents play with children's toes and fingers, and the excitement was contagious. Looking back on it, she thought he had plenty to be excited about; very few people had ever seen this kind of thing before, and he must have known that they were at the eve of making a kind of history.

The visits began to take on a new pattern. While still holding her fingers, Dr. Trentham next would bend down closer and say, "Look, there are hairs on your hand again!" as though he had found gold.

Cynthia would laugh and say, "Ooh, goodie!"

And he'd say, "Gosh, you're doing *great*!" and they would both laugh at the same time.

One of the biggest milestones was when he greeted her with an impish grin and said, "No offense, but you're getting wrinkles back in your face."

During the worst of her disease she had had a perfect, pristine, wrinkle-free, Phyllis Diller face; the relaxing of the mask was among the most visible signs that she was coming back to life. Wrinkles aren't among the things most women pray for, but Cynthia knew what they meant, and she happily replied, "I'll take them."

The ultimate proof of her recovery, however, was not something that could be seen, or that most of the people in her life even knew about. After weeks of frustrating failure, one day she went into Trentham's office and announced triumphfully, "You know what? I can whistle!"

He looked at her questioningly, perhaps even worried, as though wondering if this were the sign of some untoward new development in her disease. "You can what?"

She puckered up and demonstrated. It wasn't an impressive sound, barely better than a chirp, but still distinctly what she said it was, a whistle. As people are losing their lives to disease, there are certain things some of them keep track of as benchmarks of their own, not the capacity of the heart or lungs or their responses to stress, but the small things that tell them they're alive. One of those small things Cynthia had lost to her scleroderma was the ability to whistle. When she began getting better, it was something she would test herself for, and for many long months she would fail.

In those attempts she would do awful things to her face, scrunching it up with both hands, puffing out her cheeks, trying to make the skin loose enough that she could get back the flexibility in her lips. One day after going through this exercise, to her amazement a sound came out. It was one of the greatest moments of her life.

After the one-note demonstration in Dr. Trentham's office, now that she had his attention and in the hope of improving her musical output in an encore performance, she again pummeled and contorted her face, pursing and pulling at her lips, kneading the still unsupple skin, and tried again. This time she produced a very credible "Shave and a haircut, two bits," followed by a deep, exultant bow.

"Why are you doing that?" he asked in puzzled admiration. "Do you have a dog?"

"No," she said, laughing, "it's just one of those things I wanted to be able to do again."

"I'm going to write about it," he said, still shaking his head. But he was laughing as well.

The day finally came when Dr. Trentham told her she was in remission. She looked up the word when she got home, and although it wasn't necessarily the same thing as a cure, at least it meant they had apparently stopped her unstoppable disease.

In the summer of 1995, he took her off the minocycline. She found herself thinking, "Okay, the day I stop the medication my body is going to stay the same," but in the back of her mind that wasn't what was going to happen at all; she had lived so long with the inevitability of death, she could not rid herself of the fear that with the termination of the magic elixir, she would start sliding backward into the pit.

Dr. Trentham was watching her closely for any sign at all of the same thing, but it didn't happen. Instead, to their mutual astonishment, she just kept getting better. Even after stopping the medicine, every time Cynthia went for a check-up she would show him some new improvement. When she had stopped the minocycline, she still had residual brownish areas scattered across her skin, and they continued to diminish and finally disappeared entirely; the coloring returned to normal and her skin looked completely healthy again. Another benchmark was her hands. The contractures had already begun to loosen, but even after she stopped the antibiotic they continued to improve to the point where she was able to lay both hands flat again, something she hadn't been able to do for years. Dr. Trentham referred to what happened after they turned off the medicine as a spontaneous healing.

Even though Cynthia knew she was in remission, she still would wake up in the morning and lie there listening to her body, and if she detected a little tingling or a sensation of some kind, she would sit on the edge of her bed and think to herself that it was coming back. Now that may be behind her. She went to her family doctor a week before our second meeting, and after looking at her chart he told her, "It says you're cured of your disease." A couple of days later I had called from Ohio and, not realizing she would consider it news, I mentioned that Dr. Trentham had said the same thing. "I've been feeling like a little kid again," she said at the end of our interview.

No one has enough experience with the treatment to know how long to wait before deciding a remission is a cure. Either way, Dr. Trentham has assured her that even if it were to return at some time in the future, they already have established that minocycline works, so at the worst it would only mean that she had to go back on the therapy until it remits again.

Five years after her diagnosis, three years after she started getting better, and two years after stopping all medication, with nearly all the signs of her disease behind her, Cynthia will still sometimes whistle while walking down that long hallway by her office.

She does it because she is alive. And because she is able to.

312- 695-2344
N Weston
Promote to Leg

## CHAPTER ELEVEN

# Pinch Me

James Freeman graduated with a BSEE from Howard University in Washington in 1965, married a classmate named Phyllis Barbour a year later, then served four years in the Air Force which included a year and a half of graduate study in aerospace management sciences at the University of Southern California. He left the service with the rank of captain, and while Phyllis went on to the University of Pennsylvania for a masters in psychiatric social work and then Hunter College for her doctorate in program design and evaluation, he threw himself headlong into the challenge of beginning a career. Like many other natural entrepreneurs who come up to the starting line armed with a science education in a time of exploding technology, his subsequent path carried him far beyond the original focus of his education. He has started and done well in a variety of business ventures, ranging from consulting to the manufacture of precast tunnel liners.

Two decades later, toward the end of 1988, Phyllis pointed out to him one morning that his skin, normally a light brown, seemed to be darkening. Neither of them was particularly concerned with physical appearances but Jim said he had noticed it as well and had wondered at first if it were just his imagination. Now, when he looked in the mirror, they decided that his lips appeared to be more affected than elsewhere, taking on a deep, unhealthy shade of purple. Standing behind him, Phyllis next said that there was a reverse anomaly, where the skin was becoming lighter, in a thin border along the hairline just above the back of his neck.

Jim thought briefly of going to see a doctor, but the problem seemed trivial, an issue more of vanity than health. Besides, his life was full to brimming. He had a terrific marriage, their two children were excelling in school, his business interests were doing well, and his wife's career was right on track. He reminded himself that his grandmother, Ma Riley, had lived to be 107, and in the absence of any symptoms of illness such as pain or fatigue, he shrugged at the changes and focused instead on the far more interesting process of stewarding his talents and his blessings.

In 1991, he noticed a new development, still subtle but decidedly more ominous. He felt a constriction in the skin around his neck as though the collar of his shirt was buttoned too tightly, even when he wasn't wearing a shirt or when it wasn't buttoned at all.

The Freemans were living in New Hampshire at the time, and Jim saw a doctor in Nashua who took X-rays of his back and neck. The pictures showed a slight arthritic deterioration in the bone structure. Jim told him about his skin, but apparently because of the X-rays the doctor remained focused on the bones. He said there was nothing to worry about, that the problem was just a part of growing old. Jim, who was barely fifty, thought again of Ma Riley and wondered why he would show these early signs of aging while he had still not lived half the number of her many years. The doctor sent him to a physical therapist with the goal of working out the tightness and restoring some of his earlier flexibility.

Over the following months, Jim's business began taking him with increasing frequency to Texas, and he finally moved his family there in early 1993.

He had barely arrived when he began to experience new trouble, this time in his hands. He couldn't flex the fingers as easily as before, and it felt as though the condition in his neck had somehow migrated to the ends of his arms. He played golf a lot, and like any good duffer, his first impulse was to try correcting the problem by a change in equipment. But increasing the diameter in the handle of his clubs didn't help; in addition to the stiffness, his grip seemed to be weakening, and after observing the phenomenon for a few weeks, he decided he was beginning to lose strength and muscle tone. Clearly, it was time to get another professional opinion.

The next doctor was a young, African-American internist named Dr. Rita Phillips. After giving him a complete physical, she told him she wasn't sure but that she suspected possible involvement with his immune system. First, however, she wanted to eliminate the possibility of carpal tunnel syndrome, and referred him to a group clinical practice in Dallas specializing in that condition. They ran some tests which proved negative, but the visit was worthwhile anyway. Two of the new doctors commented on the slick, unnatural shininess to the skin of his arms, and after they consulted with each other briefly, they told him that he had some of the symptoms of a disease called scleroderma.

When Dr. Phillips got their report, she sent Jim to a rheumatologist named Susan Comer, who examined him thoroughly, did some blood work, and confirmed the diagnosis, all in one visit. Dr. Comer also pointed out that his skin, especially on the arms and neck in the areas where it had become slick and shiny, had started to harden.

Jim learned the name of his disease in the summer of 1993. By then, his hands were continually swollen and the discoloration in the hairline which his wife first had noticed five years before in New Hampshire had begun migrating from the back border of his scalp toward the front as well, forming the start of a light, unnatural halo. A similar phenomenon was appearing around his nails and fingertips—a blanching of the skin which was all the more pronounced for the contrast with the darkening elsewhere.

Now that Jim knew he was seriously ill—that indeed his disease was considered fatal—he often found himself pondering the limits of his education. Like most people, he had made a point of learning those things he thought he would need to know in life, at first related to engineering, then later to other aspects of business relevant to whatever new enterprise caught his interest. But in all the years he had been in school, he now reflected, he had never taken a single course in the human body. He knew little beyond the rudiments of anatomy, and almost nothing about physiology, the immune system, biology, or the process of disease. His children, Kimberly, twenty-five, and David, twenty-three, were used to their father knowing just about everything he needed to know in the areas that directly affected their lives, and they dealt with their own misgivings for the future by gently joking with him about the turn of events in which he so suddenly had found himself to be both vulnerable and ignorant.

Dr. Comer was candid in admitting there wasn't much she could offer in the way of help or hope, but she put Jim on a schedule of office visits every ninety days for blood work and a physical examination so she could closely monitor the progress of the disease. She also referred him to other specialists to check his lungs, liver, kidneys, stomach and other internal organs known to be common scleroderma targets. And she strongly encouraged him to stop smoking, which he did immediately.

By the time of the seventh or eighth visit, near the start of 1995, he began to experience difficulties with his digestive system, including reflux, bloatedness, diarrhea, and an uncomfortable burning sensation in his stomach. He was five-foot-eleven, and his normal weight was around two hundred pounds, but in just a few months he dropped down to 182. By itself, the weight loss might not have been a bad thing, but along with the discomfort, he also noticed a decline in strength and flexibility, enough to make him suspect that the weight change was principally the result of a loss of muscle.

The first and only medication Dr. Comer prescribed was Prilosec, a delayed-release capsule whose principal ingredient is a compound that inhibits the secretion of gastric acids. She acknowledged that the digestive problems were most likely secondary to his disease, but she never prescribed any form of treatment specifically for the scleroderma.

Any disease with an unknown etiology and no effective therapy is a natural subject of speculation as to its cause, and Jim frequently thought back to events and environments in his life prior to the onset of symptoms. One of his best suspects, if not to the cause at least to its trigger, had to do with the plant near Cleveland, Ohio, which he visited frequently several years earlier while consulting on the Los Angeles Transit System.

The product that brought him there was made of rubber bonded to an aluminum post with powerful adhesives. The factory also produced a number of other extruded rubber items, and every time he went there in 1988 and throughout most of 1989, the strong, acrid odor would creep into his sinuses and down his throat, even permeating his clothing so when he left the building it got into his car and he took it home with him. He thought of the smell at the time primarily as a tolerable annoyance; everyone knew that working with rubber was a lot like working with fish or making paper, that an odor came with the territory and was just one of those things you have to get used to. But in reflecting on it later, he recalled that occasionally he had wondered—idly, and without the kind of focus that results in action— whether it also might represent a potential hazard to his health.

The Prilosec controlled the stomach problems, but meanwhile the other aspects of his disease continued to worsen. He experienced a further decline in his energy, his appetite, and his sex drive, and occasionally now his mouth would become dry, as though the salivary glands were declining in productivity and threatening to shut down. Because he had increasing difficulty controlling the movement of his lips, his word formation was slower; sometimes he slurred his speech, and so he became more deliberate, even at times plodding, in the way he spoke.

One day when Phyllis met him at the airport after a business trip, she complained that she could hardly understand a word he was saying to her. "It's my scleroderma," he replied dejectedly. "The muscles and skin around my mouth are getting so tight, I can hardly talk."

She looked at him with mock reproach. "Jim, I do not believe that's scleroderma. You may be having some difficulty with your muscles, but I think the real problem is that you've gotten lazy."

He returned the look uncertainly, then began to smile.

"Now I'm going to give you just five seconds to repeat what you just said, and this time I expect to understand every word."

He laughed, and tried again. This time, with a little extra effort, the answer came out perfectly.

During each of his periodic visits, Dr. Comer examined Jim's skin, drew blood, and questioned him on how he felt. Frequently she would take photographs of his face and limbs, to develop a pictorial record as the changes in pigment and skin texture progressed upward along his arms and legs, and the band of demelanization crept further into his scalp and spread from the back of his hairline to complete the circle around the top of his head.

Although the Freemans discussed his disease within their immediate family, they were guarded about his condition with others, partly to protect their privacy in a time when they were still coming to terms with the changes it was creating, and partly because they didn't want to cause alarm or undue fear among their other relatives, friends, or associates. On one occasion, Jim's mother-in-law noticed the shininess of his forearms and the tightened, leatherized look of the skin, and she asked him if he had been to a doctor. He was able to answer without telling her more than he thought it would be fair for her to have to handle. That strategy pertained in other relationships as well; if people commented on his changing appearance, they got some kind of a responsive answer, neither so cryptic as to raise doubts nor so detailed as to cause alarm. The name of the disease, or that the condition was a disease at all, remained their secret.

He heard about the Boston study in the fall of 1995. After the examination in his quarterly visit, Dr. Comer told him she had learned of an interesting new clinical trial at Beth Israel Hospital, and that it might be something for him to consider. He had appreciated the logic of her strategy up to that point in never proposing any form of treatment for the scleroderma, so this new suggestion that something could be done that might actually help his disease, even if it were still experimental, piqued his interest. With her patient's permission, Dr. Comer called Boston and spoke with the rheumatologist, an Australian woman at Harvard Medical School on a research fellowship under Dr. David Trentham, who was in charge of the scleroderma project.

Dr. Christine Le wasn't looking for any more test subjects, but she received the call with interest. The original design for the study specified ten participants, and it was already full. However, by the time of the call she knew the subject who had been diagnosed with cancer wasn't expected to live through to completion. Moreover, diffuse scleroderma was known to occur with far greater frequency among African-Americans than in other groups, and a higher percentage had been shown to have antibodies associated with diffuse skin changes. This new candidate represented an eleventh-hour opportunity to improve the racial balance and statistical relevance of the trial while bringing it back up to its initial design complement.

Because both Dr. Comer and Dr. Phillips had always been forthcoming about the prognosis for his disease, Jim had no illusions about the possible efficacy of any therapy then available, or about "getting lucky" with a spontaneous remission. Indeed, in many ways his reaction to the diagnosis followed the pattern of adaptation to impending death described in the classic work of Dr. Elisabeth Kübler-Ross, starting with denial followed by a long period of clinical depression. Phyllis and their children were aware of that pattern, and they were convinced that a person's health, even while coping with a fatal disease, could be dramatically influenced by environment, especially the attitude of friends and immediate family. Phyllis changed his diet to eliminate fried foods and to accommodate his worsening lactose intolerance, but that was only part of the family's adjustment. "We knew that in any situation involving a potentially fatal disease," she said later, "the battle is in the mind as well as the body."

Fortunately, by the time the scleroderma presented itself, both children were grown, which made it easier as well. David had been a senior at Georgetown University when his father was diagnosed, and after a year of community service he entered a program of doctoral studies in history and literature at Duke

University. Kimberly, a graduate of the University of Maryland, was working in the Smithsonian's Museum of African-American History in the Washington suburb of Anacostia. From the start, they and their mother determined to provide the most positive, upbeat environment for helping their husband and father meet his challenge. They treated him not as someone who was dying but as a special person whom they loved dearly, and they held up his spirits in every possible way.

The positive attitude they created and nurtured helped Jim deal with the steady attrition in his appearance, his muscle tone, and his energy, and helped offset the erosion in his natural spirit from the progress of the disease. There is no doubt that it also contributed to his being able to recognize the possibilities, however unlikely or remote, that lay in this new situation in Boston. He discussed it with both Dr. Comer and Dr. Phillips and with his family, and, in early January of 1996, Jim flew to Logan Airport and took a taxi across the city to Beth Israel Hospital.

Dr. Le, who turned out to be a very pretty and surprisingly young-looking woman of Vietnamese birth, greeted her new patient warmly with a somewhat incongruous "Down Under" accent and introduced him to her equally friendly and attentive mentor, a trim, red-bearded, soft-spoken, highly personable Southerner named Dr. David Trentham.

On that first meeting Dr. Le took the time to methodically examine Jim and to explain his disease in considerably more detail than he had heard before. In particular, she emphasized the importance of closely monitoring his blood pressure, telling him that if a problem with hypertension arose and was detected in time it could easily be corrected, but that if it were allowed to go unnoticed or untreated, the combination with scleroderma could soon become fatal. By now Jim had a lot of experience in how people dealt with the terminal nature of his disease, and he was impressed that like Dr. Phillips and Dr. Comer, she had a talent for directness without ever creating alarm.

She also explained the nature of the study and its purpose, which was to examine the impact, if any, the antibiotic minocycline might have on his disease. She told him what he already knew about there being no standard therapy for scleroderma, and that although some doctors chose to treat their patients with one or another of the arthritis medicines, none had been shown to offer any significant long-term benefit. She said there were other studies of potential medicines for scleroderma from time to time, and that one was currently underway at Boston University Medical School on a treatment called photophoresis. She mentioned that photophoresis had been examined before without success, and she remained carefully neutral about the possibility that any of the studies or treatments, including her own, would produce a positive result. Because of its rarity, she said, scleroderma was an orphan disease, and the pharmaceutical industry and the government lacked the incentive to invest in a major research effort.

Jim began the minocycline therapy during that first visit, and set a schedule for his return at ninety-day intervals over the course of the coming forty-eight weeks.

On his second trip to Boston, Dr. Le asked him if he would be willing to participate just a couple of weeks later in a presentation on scleroderma at Beth Israel by a leading specialist in that disease whose practice included a number of African-Americans in Alabama. He agreed, and on his return toward the end of that month he found himself the focus of intense interest by the specialist and a group of internists who interviewed him at great length about his illness. Dr. Trentham attended as well. He pointed out certain aspects such as the progressive loss of pigmentation around his scalp and fingers, the darkening elsewhere, and other skin changes which were characteristics of scleroderma, and he amplified on the significance of some of the other symptoms, as well as the changes which Jim reported to be experiencing since the start of minocycline therapy. Probably most convincing to the doctors was the fact that his skin scores had dropped from 15 at the first visit to 6 just ninety days later.

For the patient, participating in this kind of event has the same negative potential impact on the spirit as being the guest of honor at an autopsy, and Jim was glad Trentham was there; his obvious caring and compassion, treating him first and foremost as a human being whose body contained information that could be of use to others, set a tone of courtesy and careful gratitude from which the meeting never wavered.

Halfway through the study, in the summer of 1996, Jim knew that a new business commitment would require him to leave Texas soon, so he went to see Dr. Comer at her office in Dallas for what would be his final visit. She made no attempt to disguise her astonishment and delight at the improvements that had taken place in his appearance, and on his way home he reflected on the contrast with what he had felt just three years before, when he had left her office with a death sentence. Not only had his spirits improved along with the rest of his condition, but he kept thinking of what might have happened if Dr. Phillips had sent him to some other specialist, or if either physician had ever given into a conventional, pragmatic, hopeless view of his disease and had simply written him off. Without their persistence, open-mindedness, and steady positivism, it was unlikely he ever would have heard of the Harvard study, and even more remote that he would have been encouraged by any other physician to become a part of it. He thanked God for both of them.

Because he was the last patient to enter the study, he was also the last to complete it, and by then Dr. Le's fellowship had come to an end and she had returned to Australia. Jim's final appointment at Beth Israel was further delayed by the chaos of relocating his family to the Washington suburb of Reston, Virginia, and so he didn't get back up to Boston until early spring of 1997.

The new doctor was another research fellow, Dr. Alejandro Morales, and as he conducted the exit examination which completed the study, he repeatedly expressed satisfaction bordering on open astonishment at the apparent results. There was much to marvel at. During the months since the therapy began, Jim's skin had become softer and more pliant. The earlier tight, polished-leather quality which had accrued over the prior years had disappeared, and the color changes had begun to reverse as well.

Dr. Morales said he didn't know how many other people Jim had met who also had scleroderma, but that Jim certainly didn't look like someone with the disease. From what the young doctor knew about the rest of the study, he told Jim, most of the other people in it had responded in pretty much the same way.

As though to emphasize his point, Morales held Jim's right forearm in his left hand and compressed and released the skin between his thumb and forefinger. It wrinkled and then restored in response to the gentle pinch with a natural resiliency which would have been impossible just a few months before. The physician looked up at his patient, smiling, and pinched him again.

Jim Freeman laughed.

## CHAPTER TWELVE

# Study Results

In his 1988 autobiography, *A Taste of My Own Medicine* (later a movie with William Hurt in the lead role), rheumatologist Edward E. Rosenbaum described the dilemma that confronted him when he was writing a text on rheumatic diseases and came to scleroderma. "I was tempted to describe it in only one sentence: 'Scleroderma: we don't know the cause and we don't have the treatment.'" But he knew that wouldn't sell, so he settled for writing about theory.

Most doctors who have faced the same challenge before and since have solved it the same way. If they go so far as to match the theory with specific therapies, the text almost inevitably concludes with expressions of failure, bewilderment, and disappointment.

Five years after Rosenbaum's book, for example, Drs. Perez and Kohn reported in the *Journal of the American Academy of Dermatology* that "No standard drug or combination of drugs has been of value for ss [systemic scleroderma] in adequately controlled prospective trials." They described the record of anti-inflammatories and corticosteroids as "disappointing," citing high toxicity and the associated risk of renal failure. Work with rats suggested that the use of the immunosuppressant cyclosporine could actually accelerate the disease process in the skin and lead to kidney collapse. The record with immunomodifiers such as plasmapheresis was "discouraging," and improvement with extracorporeal photochemotherapy was "limited." They reported that "significant morbidity and mortality" were associated with the use of d-penicillamine, and that various short-term studies of colchicine were "discouraging." Of the other drugs commonly prescribed for scleroderma such as dimethyl sulfoxide (DMSO), potassium aminobenzoic acid, aspirin and dipyridamole, ketanserin, dextran, and ketotifen, they said that only one—captopril, which can reverse hypertension in patients experiencing kidney collapse—had been shown to alter the course of the disease.

As Tom Brown said more than once, you can't cure a disease without first knowing its cause. But while his prime suspect for scleroderma was an L-form microbe, most likely a mycoplasma, he also recognized that whatever infectious agent lay at the cause of this particular disease, it didn't operate in a vacuum. A lot of diseases of the connective tissue are triggered by a similar event to the one involving Pat Ganger's twisted ankle on Pelee Island, not necessarily an accident, but perhaps childbirth or the loss of a job or a shock such as the death of a friend or family member. Beyond that triggering event, there is a growing body of evidence that environment may also play a major role in the etiology of most—or all—such diseases.

A couple of years ago, public health researchers found the incidence of rheumatic disease among the permanent population on Pelee Island was 49.5 percent, or about ten times higher than the North

American average. They also discovered that the longer a resident lived there the worse the odds, with the probability of affliction five times higher among people with ten years or more in residence. Pat Ganger had been going to the island for only two years at the time of her diagnosis, but when she thought back on it, she realized she had been working with strong chemicals in the printing business for the previous eight, so her environment in that decade may have had some consistent characteristics that were equal to having spent the whole period on an island in the middle of what had once been one of the world's most polluted lakes. In many ways, she reflected later, the situation on Pelee Island matched those experienced by the similarly insular population of Allegheny County (see Chapter 2) in Pennsylvania.

Tom Brown's theory about the role of mycoplasmas in connective tissue diseases, at least as controversial as his use of minocycline therapy, received a dramatic boost in late 1996, seven-and-a-half years after his death. A report in the British medical publication *Lancet* by a group of doctors at Hospital Pellegrin in Bordeaux, France, described the isolation of a species called *mycoplasma fermentans* from the synovial lining tissues of patients with rheumatoid arthritis. In the past couple of decades, lots of such reports had been published in support of Dr. Brown's widely disputed initial claim prior to World War II, but until now their common Achilles' heel, like Brown's, had been the lack of a provable connection with the host. What made this one newsworthy was that it was the first to use the state-of-the-art PCR (polymerase chain reaction) assay, the DNA "fingerprinting" technique which gained so much public attention in the O. J. Simpson murder trial. While it still stopped short of demonstrating cause and effect, it was proof positive that Dr. Brown's suspect was at the scene of the crime.

A next logical step would be to run the same PCR assay on the biopsied skin samples of patients with scleroderma.

The clinical portion of the Harvard study was completed with James Freeman's final visit to Beth Israel in the spring of 1997. By then Dr. Christine Le had returned to Australia, so Dr. Morales and Dr. Trentham packed up the last of the data and shipped it to Melbourne. Because Australia is on both the other side of the world and the other side of the clock, the back-and-forth coordination of the results was protracted, but by mid-November Trentham's office produced a draft report entitled "Minocycline in Early Diffuse Scleroderma: A Pilot Open 12-month Study in 11 Patients."

The report said that all other medications that might potentially modify scleroderma (whether or not they ever had) were discontinued during the course of the study and required a one-month washout period. These agents included penicillamine, methotrexate, cyclosporin, cyclophosphidamide, chlorambucil, colchicine, and photophoresis. Skin biopsies were performed on all patients on enrollment. All visits included a complete history, physical examination, complete blood count, electrolytes, urea and creatinine, liver function tests, erythrocyte sedimentation rate (ESR Westergren method) and urinalysis. Serum was also collected at all visits and stored at -70°C for adhesion molecule (intracellular adhesion molecule 1 [ICAM-1], vascular cell adhesion molecule 1 [VCAM-1], and E-selectin) assays.

In order to avoid possible dizziness or headaches, which are sometimes reported by rheumatoid arthritis patients when they are started on higher doses, drug administration began with 50 mg capsules bid, with water on an empty stomach, then increased to 100 mg after the first month. Patients were instructed to stay away from milk or other dairy products, antacids, and any medicines or supplements with iron.

Skin scores were measured at each visit, and a response was not counted as clinically significant unless it showed a decrease of more than 35 percent by the last examination. The researchers used a patient and physician 10-cm visual analog scale (VAS) to measure global patient status, where 0 cm meant the patient could not be better, and 10 cm could not be worse; a clinically significant response was defined as a decrease of at least 25 percent in twelve months.

All eleven patients enrolled in the study, coming from six states and Canada, had been diagnosed by at least one independent rheumatologist. Six of the subjects were referred by rheumatologists, and five came through The Road Back Foundation.

At the end of the year, five patients had dropped out of the study, two because of a renal crisis (from the disease, not the medicine) just two months after entry, two for noncompliance with the protocol, and one because of death from a pre-existing cancer which was not detected until after the study began. In the two cases of renal crisis, neither was taking angiotensin-converting enzyme inhibitors during the study; afterward, one returned to normal while the other required permanent dialysis. One of the two non-compliers stopped minocycline after nine months because she felt it wasn't working, although her skin score at six months was 60 percent better than at enrollment. The other noncomplier quit the study in order to switch over to intravenous minocycline therapy. Three of the dropouts were due to serious intercurrent morbidity.

Six patients completed the full course of treatment.

In all, nine of the eleven patients in the study (82 percent) experienced significant improvement in skin scores. At the end of one year, four of them had complete resolution of their skin disease and their final skin scores were zero; in three of those four, patient and physician VAS scores had improved to zero as well.

Scleroderma could be cured.

## CHAPTER THIRTEEN

# Is It Safe?

Does the question sound familiar?

Millions of moviegoers remember it as the sinister, oft-repeated query by the fugitive Nazi physician played by Sir Laurence Olivier in *Marathon Man*. Every time the White Angel asks Dustin Hoffman's young student, "Is it safe?" none of us thinks for a minute that it is out of any concern for the well-being of his intended victim. Quite the contrary, the evil doctor, up from the jungles of Paraguay to cash in his trove of stolen diamonds, hardly expects the Hoffman character to live through dinner.

This same question illuminates one of those areas of medicine in which life frequently imitates art. In evaluating risk versus benefit, physicians always weigh the perils to themselves as well as to the patient, and if there is a conflict, the patient's interests usually will come in second. Regardless of how many times a standard therapy has been proven worthless or even downright dangerous, it's still a lot safer *for the doctor* than prescribing any modality that has not yet gained acceptance in a particular application. It equally doesn't matter how many times a therapy may have been applied successfully in an off-label use, or even if it has demonstrated the potential for saving the patient's life. Their own professional security is the sole reason that some of the same doctors who consider tetracycline safe enough to prescribe for millions of adolescents with nothing more serious than pimples will unblushingly question its safety in the treatment of a disease that can, and usually does, kill.

Dr. Thomas McPherson Brown was an exception. Over the course of his long career he prescribed the off-label use of antibiotics to some ten thousand patients with connective tissue disease. He knew as well as everyone else in medicine that tetracyclines are famous for their benign profile, and he stated in *The Road Back* that he had "not seen any toxic effects in forty years in anybody." Nor did one of those many patients ever complain of a single instance of malpractice or misfeasance. Indeed, dermatologist Alan R. Cantwell, Jr., who studied the infectious etiology of scleroderma and lupus for more than a quarter century, recently described antibiotic therapy as "far safer than steroids, aspirin, non-steroidal anti-inflammatory agents, gold, and methotrexate."

While antibiotics in general have the disadvantage of often encouraging resistant strains of the diseases they attack, tetracyclines are almost uniquely disinclined to that result. The reason is that the decision to resist is formed in the wall of an organism, not in its core, and the bugs that this class of antibiotic most precisely targets are so-called cell-wall deficient organisms such as mycoplasmas, where the means for a resistance response are poorly formed or nonexistent.

Tetracyclines, in common with any other medicine, can sometimes have side effects, but beyond sun-sensitivity during the course of therapy and occasional vaginal yeast infections in women (easily corrected with nothing more drastic than a small helping of yogurt), adverse responses are rare and few. The antibiotic can cause transient dizziness and stomach queasiness, and occasional discoloration of the skin and, in young children, of the teeth. More serious reactions such as hypersensitivity syndrome reaction, serum sickness, and what has been described as a drug-induced form of lupus, occur with such minuscule frequency that they collectively amount to a tiny fraction of one percent of the number of the far more deadly complaints associated with non-steroidal anti-inflammatory drugs (NSAIDs) alone. There are contraindications for the use of any medicine, but most practitioners, like Cantwell, "have never heard of anyone becoming seriously ill with tetracycline, or even minocycline."

The claim that tetracyclines are safer than any of the other therapies is more than a figure of speech. Conventional treatments for rheumatoid arthritis (frequently prescribed for scleroderma even though they produce no measurable long-term benefit) can often be more devastating than the affliction they purport to treat. In late 1988, *Newsweek* ran a cover story on the recent finding by the Food and Drug Administration that non-steroidal anti-inflammatory drugs, prescribed primarily for rheumatoid arthritis, caused "silent ulcers" which were killing up to twenty thousand Americans a year. That was considerably more people than the number then believed to die annually from arthritis, and was equal to the mortality estimates for the far rarer scleroderma. NSAIDs were reformulated that same year and the losses were cut by an estimated 85 percent, but that "more acceptable" level still leaves a death rate equal to the crash of a fully loaded jumbo jet once every month.

For another comparison, consider Pat Ganger's experience with d-penicillamine. Although her initial response to the drug was that in the first year it seemed to help with the soreness and produced a slight loosening of the skin, those benefits proved transitory. It was well established that penicillamine can cause problems with blood cell production in the bone marrow, but with the continued hardening of her skin, that risk became impossible to monitor. Moreover, up to the time she stopped treatment after five years of ineffectual therapy, not a single placebo-controlled, double-blind clinical study of this drug had ever been conducted to determine whether it was worth doing in the first place. When such trials finally were completed on penicillamine in scleroderma some eight years after Pat had quit, they simply proved what she and many others knew already: the drug did virtually nothing to halt the long-term progress of the disease.

Let's look at methotrexate, which was initially developed to battle cancer. *The Road Back* cites a 1987 study conducted at McMaster University in Ontario by Tugwell, Bennett, and Gent of the efficacy and safety of this drug in the treatment of rheumatoid arthritis. It reported nausea, vomiting, anorexia, and diarrhea in 10 percent of the subjects surveyed; stomatitis (inflammatory disease of the mouth) in 6 percent; leukopenia (low production of white blood cells), anemia, or thrombocytopenia (another blood deficiency normally associated with hemorrhage) in 3 percent; and "rare" instances of toxicity of the liver, kidneys, or lungs, possible malignancy, reduced sperm production in males, excessive development of male breasts, fever, localized osteoporosis, and another blood/arterial complication called leukocytonbastic vasculitis. Although therapy had to be discontinued in one-third of those surveyed because of these and other effects, the authors concluded that, "If approved [by the FDA], the drug should be given to patients with rheumatoid arthritis refractory to first- and second-line agents, such as injectable gold and penicillamine, who provide informed consent." Despite all these setbacks and even though methotrexate has never produced a single provable long-term benefit to arthritis patients in the decade since that study, it has become rheumatology's drug of choice in the treatment of severe rheumatoid arthritis.

Of course they're already using it on scleroderma. Last year, the *British Journal of Rheumatology* published the results of a double-blind study of twenty-nine patients in the Netherlands, seventeen of whom started off on 15 milligrams of injectable methotrexate once a week for twenty-four weeks and twelve patients getting a placebo. During the observational phase, also twenty-four weeks, which followed, the placebo group had the option of switching over to the drug, and nonresponders in the methotrexate group were allowed to increase their weekly dose to 25 milligrams. There were thirteen adverse reactions, withdrawals, or deaths reported within the study period, and all but two of them were in the group receiving methotrexate. Six temporarily withdrew because of liver problems, all of them on the drug. One more withdrew permanently because of violent headaches from the drug, and another due to renal crisis related to the disease. One placebo patient withdrew because of renal crisis as well. There were three deaths: one in each group was related to scleroderma, and the third, in the methotrexate group, is believed to have resulted from a heart attack.

Aside from that, the good news is that more than two-thirds of the methotrexate patients demonstrated an improvement of 30 percent or better in skin thickness or general well-being and without further damage to internal organs. But like penicillamine, there is no evidence that these changes are more than symptomatic or that they significantly outlast the patient's tolerance to the medication.

This chapter opened with a memory test, so let's close it the same way. How many of us can recall thalidomide? Even if you weren't around when this sedative/hypnotic first appeared on the scene a generation ago, you probably recognize the name as a paradigm for the unthinkable. Although thalidomide was never officially approved by the FDA, large amounts of the drug were brought into this country for personal use by visitors returning from the United Kingdom, where it was available in pharmacies by prescription. Some of those travelers, or their friends in America with whom they shared this forbidden apple, were women, and some of those women were pregnant.

But—was it safe?

Britons found out the answer before we did, because they started using thalidomide sooner. At first the horrific results were kept quiet, but even if they had been disclosed immediately it wouldn't have made that much difference. By the time the public realized they had bitten into a worm, it was too late. Thousands of expectant mothers on both sides of the Atlantic who had taken the drug to help them get to sleep, including some who had used it only once or twice, gave birth to malformed babies, some without eyes or ears, many with limbs that were severely truncated or missing entirely. Uncounted thousands more elected to end their pregnancies, some on the knowledge that the fetus was malformed, and some simply on the risk that it might be. It was one of the most tragic mass poisonings in the history of medicine.

Even if the general public doesn't have a terrific collective memory, we can be sure the pharmaceutical industry hasn't forgotten its experience with thalidomide any more than Union Carbide is likely to forget Bhopal or Exxon will forget the Valdez disaster. However, it has been observed that history, like character, is not determined by triumphs or calamities alone, but by what happens next. And what is happening next with the admirably resilient industry that brought us thalidomide the first time? They're bringing it back.

As of this writing, volunteers are being sought through notices in hospitals, medical journals, letters, and on the Internet to participate in a new twelve-week therapeutic study of this drug in the United States. "All women of child-bearing age must have a negative pregnancy test at the screening and must practice effective contraception for at least one month prior to study entry," the call specifies, "with at least two forms of birth control (an oral or implanted contraceptive and a barrier method) while part of the study. During the study, all women in this age group will receive biweekly pregnancy tests."

These days the drug isn't being tested for how well it helps women get to sleep, but on whether it does anything useful for scleroderma.

"Why on earth would anyone test a drug on our disease when it is already known to have such terrible side effects?" one scleroderma patient asked when she heard about the thalidomide study. "Do they think most of us are too young to remember? Or have they decided that as a group, because we're probably going to die anyway, we represent a different level of risk?"

## CHAPTER FOURTEEN

# Tailoring the Therapy

The first step toward effective therapy for any disease is an accurate diagnosis. Many of the routine laboratory tests are normal for most scleroderma patients, so in the early stages before more classic symptoms have become evident, the diagnosis can be elusive. For example, about a third of all scleroderma patients test positive for rheumatoid factor, which leaves two-thirds who do not. The blood sedimentation rate, which is often a clue to other connective tissue diseases, is usually normal or just slightly elevated. A positive antinuclear antibody (ANA) is another indicator of this same class of diseases and can often, but not always, be a sign of diffuse scleroderma (anti-RNA) and limited scleroderma and polymyositis (anti-PM Scl.) There is no single blood test specifically for scleroderma, so most diagnoses depend on a combination of the above tests and the clinical observation of symptoms, sometimes including microscopic evidence of tissues obtained by biopsy.

Two methods which are helpful in monitoring the status of the disease after diagnosis are Anti-Scl-70, which measures a nuclear enzyme found in the systemic form, and such antibody tests as anti-DNA, anti-Sm, RNP, and anti-Ro to measure serum complement levels.

As for what happens next, there is a temptation in medicine, as elsewhere in life, to believe that if something is found to be good for us, more of it is even better. Sometimes that's true, and sometimes it's not. The early history of anti-inflammatories and antibiotics, for two examples, saw prescriptions written for many times the dosage levels which subsequently proved effective on the disease or even safe for the patient. More recent experience has seen the opposite.

Prednisone, which responsible physicians today dole out in 5 or 10 milligram tablets to help manage the discomfort or pain of inflammation, was initially prescribed in doses as much as eighty or a hundred times higher—and sometimes still is. By the time a patient with a connective tissue disease is no longer able to tolerate the therapy, which can happen very soon at those high levels, the prognosis is likely to be complicated by cataracts, weak, unhealthy "cortisone skin," and kidney failure. When susceptibility to any of these same problems is also a characteristic of the disease, such as skin anomalies or renal collapse in the case of scleroderma, the problem is compounded. Moreover, because the treatment of external effects can merely mask the disease without doing anything for its cause, the original problem has usually gotten far worse by the time the suppressed symptoms suddenly return with a vengeance. A prolonged heavy hand can also burn out the body's ability to manufacture anti-inflammatories on its own, so the unnatural dependency becomes permanent.

For some of the same reasons, too much of an antibiotic can create more problems than it cures. But conversely, as has been demonstrated in recent experience with Lyme disease, so can *under*prescribing either the dosage level or the duration of therapy. Choosing the right drug is only part of the solution. The development of an appropriate protocol for its administration is also important.

The way most medical protocols are established is by trial and error, by varying the parameters and observing the results, keeping track of what works and what doesn't. Regardless of what it says on the bottle, many doctors adjust dosage levels, frequencies, and even routes of administration to the needs and responses of the patient, with the ultimate goal of reducing the amount as quickly as possible and as far as possible while still controlling the disease. In the short term, the adjustment can go up or down.

In 1988, Carol Lange experienced a severe flare of rheumatoid arthritis, a disease which her doctor, Thomas McPherson Brown, had been controlling with antibiotics for the previous twenty-five years. Dr. Brown knew that flares, in common with fast-moving or severe diseases as well as all forms of scleroderma, require aggressive intervention. As usual, he started her off with 300 milligrams of clindamycin administered intravenously the first day, then 600 the second, and 900 every day for the balance of the week, along with her regular course of oral minocycline, and the flare slowly receded. (At a recent conference of physicians experienced in antibiotic therapy for scleroderma and other connective tissue diseases, there was a consensus that this combination approach was the most effective in dealing with such extremes.) But Dr. Brown died a short time later, and Carol had to find another doctor.

This time the physician was Albert Dawkins, a rheumatologist in nearby Maryland who had worked with Brown at George Washington University Medical School, first as a protégé and then as a colleague, and had developed a considerable body of his own experience in treating hundreds of arthritis patients with antibiotic therapy. He handled Carol's next flare with the same drug and at the same dosage level as were used by Brown, but with her assent and based on his success with other patients he doubled the frequency to twice a day and extended it two days longer. He also combined the antibiotic therapy with an NSAID and antihistamine, both administered orally. The approach worked so well that whenever Carol had a flareup over the following years, she and Dawkins could predict its course with nearly clockwork accuracy. At the fifth day, following her Herxheimer reaction, they would see a remarkable reduction in her pain and related disease activity, and she would walk out of the hospital, pain-free, her symptoms completely reversed, and with no disabilities at the end of the treatment.

Dr. Dawkins understood that the Jarisch Herxheimer reaction was a temporary, dose-induced flareup, and not a toxic reaction to the drug. Carol had agreed to ride out the reaction in order to achieve a long-term benefit from the elevated dosage. Among other things, finding the right combination comes down to the doctor's experience with the therapy and the patient's history and levels of tolerance.

As of this writing, most physicians have never prescribed minocycline for scleroderma, which means that some will now be looking for guidelines to that application. So far the only such published protocol is in the Harvard study. Although that's a good starting point, it is hardly written in stone. Not everyone is the same age, weight, height, race, or gender, they don't share a common immune system, and they don't have identical medical histories. Regardless of what guidelines a doctor follows for any drug, it is commonplace to adjust the parameters of dosage, frequency, term, and sometimes combinations with other medicines to the needs of each patient. For obvious reasons, such variations are not permissible in a controlled study, but in their clinical practices rheumatologists do it all the time with prednisone, Naprosyn, methotrexate, plaquinil, penicillamine, gold salts, and all the other drugs they prescribe, whether for scleroderma, rheumatoid arthritis, or some other connective tissue disease.

Less commonplace in medicine, however, is the use of antibiotics over a prolonged period of time. Although most rheumatologists are comfortable offering any of the above nostrums for as long as the patient can tolerate them before losing liver or kidney function or going blind, most schedules for the use of antibiotics in the treatment of infectious disease are no longer than a week or ten days. There's a good reason for this restraint in the use of antibiotics in general: ten days is usually long enough to do the job, and overusing them can encourage the development of resistant strains of the bugs they were designed to kill.

Scleroderma is not like most other infectious diseases, and for the reasons already discussed, minocycline is not like most other antibiotics. Tom Brown learned from his earliest experience with the elusive L-forms that they were capable of such astonishing tenacity. It was sometimes necessary to keep up the antibiotic pressure for months and even years. This was far less often the case with scleroderma, but even there it was clearly impossible to gain any lasting, measurable benefits with as brief a regimen as ten days.

During periods when the patients were hospitalized for intensive therapy, Dr. Brown concentrated the treatment for maximum impact, and for the same reasons Dr. Dawkins took an even more aggressive approach at such times. But for the maintenance programs by which this therapy was administered the rest of the time, most other experienced doctors, including Dawkins, followed Brown's technique of spacing the doses in response to the needs of the patient. At one point, Carol Lange was on a schedule of five days of medication followed by two days off, and at other times she was on every other day, every third day, or two on and one off; the most common schedule was three times a week, with nothing on Saturdays and Sundays.

The principle behind this irregular schedule was based on the fact that tetracycline will stay in the body for forty-eight hours or more after oral administration. The spacing allowed the body to rest between doses without losing the cumulative impact of the antibiotic, which is held in low-metabolizing tissues such as bones and cartilage where it can still be drawn into the system, albeit at lower levels, even on days when no drug is given. Pat Ganger recently developed a graph showing the relationship between the peaking of antibiotic activity and the subsequent peaking of antigenic activity with the use of minocycline. Daily doses create a relatively steady condition in which the minocycline might be expected to initiate a hypersensitivity reaction, while alternating doses avoids the overlapping effect and can sometimes, although not always, allow the hypersensitivity reaction to remit. Likewise, too much antibiotic at any one time can trigger a similar problem which is often relieved by nothing more complex than an adjustment in the dose.

Dr. Harold Clark says two other advantages of the pulse method are that the off days give the body tissues a respite from the oxidation associated with the use of antibiotics, as well as provide an interim for restoration of normal protein synthesis in the cells. Mycoplasmas are relatively lethargic reproducers, so any such small hiatus is unlikely to encourage a breeding spree.

One other factor to consider in the use of any drug, particularly antibiotics, is the huge differences in effectiveness which can sometimes exist between the original branded product and it generic counterpart. The FDA requires that any generic form must have a bioequivalence within 20 percent of the drug it copies, which means that two generic versions of the same drug can vary from each other by as much as 40 percent in effectiveness. This can be especially problematic in the case of minocycline, which can be chemically equivalent under the law but miss the mark altogether in terms of clinical benefits with diseases as complex as inflammatory arthritis, lupus, or scleroderma. In rheumatoid arthritis, where the body of clinical experience is far greater than with scleroderma, very often the only difference between a response and a nonresponse to minocycline is whether the prescription is filled with the original Lederle formulation, branded as Minocin, or a generic dud.

## CHAPTER FIFTEEN

# In Defense of Heresy

There's an old story about a policeman who encounters a drunk at around midnight, down on his hands and knees, searching the sidewalk under a street-lamp. When questioned, the drunk says he's looking for a silver dollar he dropped an hour earlier at the other end of the block. "So what are you doing down here?" the officer asks. "Why aren't you looking where you lost it?"

"Use your head," the searcher replies, squinting into the void beyond the ring of the streetlamp, "it's as black as the pit out there. What chance would I have of finding it in the dark?"

You can see that same joke repeated every day on every well-lighted street corner in medicine. Searchers by the thousands scour the same old territory for as long as the light lasts, in some rare cases just to prove the ground is fallow, but far more often for no better reason than the certainty that even when they come up empty-handed they still get paid for looking.

And what about the far fewer researchers who are actually willing to work in the dark where answers await discovery, the true scientists who are led by a hunch or happenstance to challenge a tradition or consensus which is always heavily defended by politics and myth? They can be assured of a very hard road: shunning or outright attacks by colleagues who frequently are also their rivals, little or no grant support, restricted access or no access to peer-reviewed media, loss of reputation, frequently loss of income, and sometimes loss of employment.

When the producer of *20/20* asked Tom Brown why he had written a book for the general public which challenged the conventional view of connective tissue disease after four decades of nearly constant attack by the medical establishment for those very same heresies, he answered with a tired smile, "Because I've finally outlived the sons of bitches." But of course, he hadn't. The real reason Tom wrote the book was because he knew he was dying. If there was any doubt of the outcome, by the time the segment aired it was abundantly apparent the sons of bitches were going to outlive the pioneer. They frequently do.

In 1984, Dr. Barry Marshall was serving out his residency at a hospital in Perth, Australia. At about the same age as Tom Brown and Albert Sabin had been when they began their careers at the Rockefeller Institute some half-century earlier, he too made a discovery that one day would revolutionize medicine. Suspecting that bacteria, not stress, were the cause of stomach ulcers, he and a colleague had taken samples from the stomachs of ulcer patients and were trying to culture something in a petri dish. The standard incubation time is forty-eight hours, and like Tom Brown with mycoplasma, they had come up empty in their first several attempts to isolate a potential culprit. By chance, over the Easter holidays, one batch was left in its dish for more than twice the normal length of time, and they returned to find a colony of corkscrew-like *Helicobacter pylori* swarming under the microscope. Repeating the technique, the same suspect appeared in cultures from other ulcer patients.

The obvious next step in Koch's postulate would be to use the bacteria to induce this disease in an animal model, as Sabin had induced arthritis with his second mouse, but those attempts proved just as unproductive as their earlier tries at culturing the bug. In frustration, young Dr. Marshall decided, perhaps rashly, to try the experiment on a human subject, swilling down a microbial cocktail which he later described as tasting like swamp water. A week later he awoke in the middle of the night with severe stomach cramps, and a few days after that an endoscopic examination with a tiny television camera revealed a gastric inflammation of the type often associated with ulcers.

Armed with these revolutionary results, Marshall hit the medical convention trail to rouse the sleeping populace—and of course his colleagues responded to the wake-up call with nudges, winks, and snickers. Who was this bothersome upstart? He came from a hospital hardly anyone had ever heard of, was still a resident, hardly even a clinician, and certainly not a researcher. Everybody knew that ulcers were caused by acid which was triggered by stress (one way of blaming the patient, as stress is usually seen as a function of lifestyle.) There had been a long-standing myth in medicine that the environment of the stomach was too hostile to support any life forms, and many doctors still adhered to that fiction even though it had been disproven before Barry Marshall ever appeared on their horizon.

Perhaps even more to the point, there was already an absolutely wonderful treatment, Tagamet, an acid-blocker approved by the FDA less than a decade earlier which had cut ulcer surgery by a third in its first year on the market and which by 1984 had become the best-selling drug on earth. From a strictly business point of view, the real magic of acid blockers was that no matter how many times they "cured" the disease, the ulcers usually came back. No investor in his right mind would want to kill the goose that lays that kind of golden annuity, and neither, apparently, would the typical gastroenterologist for whom ulcers produced a quarter of all annual income.

The more resistance he met, the more determined Dr. Marshall became. He concocted a number of different therapies aimed at knocking out both the painful symptoms and the *H. pylori* which he remained convinced was their real cause. He got a 70 percent remission rate with a combination of Pepto-Bismol and the antibiotic metronidazole, and when someone else added tetracycline to the mix the effectiveness rose another 15 points to 85 percent of all stomach ulcers treated, a number which may represent 100 percent of those with a bacterial etiology.

He also responded to the indifference or criticism of his colleagues by turning up the volume, often angrily scolding them at medical conventions about their obligation as healers to eradicate ulcers at their source, an exercise which increased his visibility in about the same degree as it reduced his peer popularity. Eventually his efforts began to attract a different constituency, and a far larger audience. After he published a paper in the British medical journal *Lancet*, the story of his work was picked up in America by *The National Enquirer*, then the *Cincinnati Enquirer*, and eventually *The Wall Street Journal*. For many, his saga became a model of everything that was wrong with how the establishment responded to innovation, how the ethics of medicine had been pre-empted by the venality of big business, and how the little guy, whether a renegade genius or a helpless patient, always gets it in the neck. It was one of the best conspiracy stories since the assassination of John F. Kennedy, only this time the victim was still alive and it looked like he finally had a chance of winning.

A decade and a half after that breakthrough in Perth, how has this process played itself out: how is Dr. Marshall viewed in the medical establishment, and how much of a difference have discovering the cause of stomach ulcers and offering an effective cure made in the way the disease is now treated?

Today it is almost universally accepted that 85 percent of all ulcers in the digestive system are caused by the bacteria he identified in 1984, and numerous clinical trials have shown that antibiotic therapy can cure them up to 100 percent of the time. Meanwhile, *H. pylori* also have been implicated in stomach cancer which, in parts of the world such as Italy and Peru where the bacteria are more ubiquitous, can be a leading cause of death. In America, the NIH have officially declared that ulcer patients with *H. pylori* should have the bacteria eradicated.

Procter & Gamble, which makes Pepto-Bismol, began supporting Dr. Marshall when they recognized that his work with bismuth against *H. pylori* might represent an opportunity to carve out a larger share in their new pharmaceutical marketplace, and under the company's powerful aegis the young renegade from Perth moved into a new position at the University of Virginia Medical School. Even though his work met with often blistering criticism, ridicule, and even personal attacks at every step of the way, almost all of his original critics have swung full circle, some gracefully and some grudgingly, in support of the infectious theory and antibiotic therapy. In 1995 he was honored by the prestigious Lasker Award for his work on ulcers, and many people consider him a prime candidate for the Nobel prize in medicine.

All of which might appear to be the happiest possible ending to these two stories, both of a truly deserving innovator and of the scourge which he has devoted his career to eradicating.

So far, that would be a false conclusion. Despite all the well-publicized evidence of its efficacy, safety, and cost-effectiveness, the number of ulcer cases actually treated by antibiotic therapy had risen only sluggishly, from zero in 1984 to a mere 16 percent in 1995, a share described by *Fortune* magazine as "amazingly few." Dr. Marshall's office at the medical school still receives panicked telephone calls from patients who are facing painful, expensive, and life-threatening surgery for a condition which the world now knows can be treated better medically, and at far less cost or risk. If the young Australian doctor ever does make it down the aisle at Oslo, it is a certainty that those plaintive calls for help will be ringing louder in his mind than anything he is likely to be hearing at the same time from his colleagues, whether their praise, their familiar but subdued snickers, or the gnashing of old teeth.

In his classic work, *The Structure of Scientific Revolutions*, the late Massachusetts Institute of Technology professor Thomas S. Kuhn sees the process previously outlined—and indeed, the process described in this book—as being not just occasional to such change, but inevitable. "Normal science," he writes, "often suppresses fundamental novelties because they are necessarily subversive of its basic commitments." He describes the major turning points in the careers of Copernicus, Newton, Lavoisier, and Einstein, among many others, as dramas in which the transforming event results not just from insight or serendipity but from the resolution of the often bitter contest between personalities, between the cultures of the status quo and the revolutionary, between deeply entrenched and heavily defended traditions that no longer work and radical changes that do, between the present and the future.

*[A] new theory, however special its range of application, is seldom or never just an increment of what is already known. Its assimilation requires the reconstruction of prior theory and the re-evaluation of prior fact, an intrinsically revolutionary process that is seldom completed by a single man and never overnight.*

That contest can be vastly more complex when the science is medicine, and the outcome of a medical revolution frequently depends far more on the strength of its champions than on the power of its truth.

Consider the case of Virginia Wuerthele-Caspe, M.D. (later and better known as Virginia Livingston-Wheeler), the lead author some years back, along with Eva Brodkin, M.D., and Camille Mermod, M.D., of a preliminary clinical report entitled "Etiology of Scleroderma." The study was based on the probable bacterial cause of scleroderma and its treatment with antibacterial agents.

"On the assumption that the organism is a mycobacterium as in leprosy and tuberculosis," she wrote, "the senior author reasoned that it should be found in nasal ulcers, subcutaneous tissue, and sputum when there is pulmonary involvement. Accordingly material was prepared from the sputum of a proved case of scleroderma. When the slides were stained by the Ziehl-Neelson method, numerous short, thick, acid-fast rods appeared." A cooperating team of investigators was formed to study the organism's pathology in six patients, all but one of whom were women.

The conclusions of the study, potentially at least, were revolutionary in the true sense of the word. "An acid-fast bacillus [was] found in five cases of scleroderma examined bacteriologically. The organism [was] found in the sputum, blood, nasal, and subcutaneous tissue smears, and has been grown in pure culture from the blood. All patients treated with promin (which destroys or inhibits mycobacteria) have shown definite, responsive changes. The organism . . . may be a newly recognized member of the family of mycobacteria."

So why isn't this book about these four muses? They were the first researchers to name mycoplasmas as the prime suspect in the disease, and the first to point directly at a scleroderma treatment that works.

In case you missed it, all three authors of the study are women, as is the researcher in charge of the lab work, a questionable advantage in medicine even in today's enlightened environment. And what they are reporting, in its context, is revolutionary, which means they are also heretics.

Because the authors were deprived of virtually all the power required for effective advocacy, their brilliant, prescient study failed to meet the acid test of What Happened Next. It was published, not in *JAMA* or *Lancet* or *Arthritis and Rheumatism*, but in *The Journal of the Medical Society of New Jersey*. It appeared in print long before the term "glass ceiling" had been coined and before "PC" meant either politically correct or personal computer, a half-century ago, in the summer of 1947. And of course, it was universally ignored.

Now, over a million scleroderma patients later, another study has been completed, this one pointing more directly to a cure for the disease; the fact that you are now reading this book means that the scientific report of that study has already been presented in a peer-reviewed medical forum. This time the revolutionary concept may have some advantage in its aegis, but it is revolutionary nonetheless and will hardly be exempted from the protracted and surely rancorous defense of the truths which it will eventually displace.

The purpose of this book is to broaden the forum in which the new truths are weighed against the old by inviting in the thousands of patients for whom this therapy can mean the difference between life and death. For doctors or patients, the experiences and insights of others who have traveled a similar road can illuminate personal choices that ease the journey.

At the bottom line, all patients are consumers, whatever the name of their disease, and they deserve not just to participate but to be in charge of the process by which they select the most appropriate therapy and hire the best physician to provide it.

## CHAPTER SIXTEEN:
# What Happened Next

This edition of *Scleroderma* follows publication of the original book by five years.

The official release date of that first edition was May 8, 1998, the same day Dr. Trentham presented the results of his study to members of the International Society for Rheumatic Therapies in Boston. That morning CNN featured the story on its main cable network, and a shorter version appeared every 15 minutes on CNN Headline News for the next four days, carrying the results to millions of viewers throughout the world.

Pat Ganger and three other directors of The Road Back Foundation (Carol Lange, Diane Aronson, and the author), attended the ISRT meeting. The media coverage assured that the story was finally going to reach the audience with the greatest need to know, an exciting payback on their long-term investment of effort, hope, and faith.

At nearly the same time as the study announcement in 1998, and coincidentally with the birth of her son, a Playboy model named Tylyn John was experiencing the first small signs that something was wrong. A year later, her symptoms included Raynaud's in her fingers, extreme fatigue, and tightening of the skin in her hands and forearms; her scleroderma was diagnosed at UCLA that summer. She was told very little about what could be done for her disease, and even less about what to expect.

Tylyn had never heard of scleroderma, and she had no recollection of the story on CNN. However, the father of one of her friends was a researcher in another branch of medicine. He began scouring the Internet for information—and with it, perhaps some badly needed hope. As Tylyn learned about her disease, she quickly decided that the standard therapies were not only ineffective, but that their effects could be worse than her symptoms. The search led her to The Road Back web site, and from there to Dr. Robert Franco, a Riverside, California, rheumatologist experienced in the antibiotic protocol.

At their first meeting in mid-December, the tightness in the skin had advanced to Tylyn's upper arms and shoulders, and was becoming evident in her mouth and cheeks. Several of her teeth began to shift position as the tissue supporting them thickened and scarred with the disease. There was also severe temporal mandibular joint involvement; she was able to open her mouth six centimeters at their first meeting, but by the following February it was down to 3.5; two months later, in response to the minocycline, it was back up to 4.6. Dr. Franco noted that Tylyn had a positive ANA (anti-nuclear antibody) test in June with a high titer of 1 in 1280. He requested the test again, and this time the titer was 1 in 640 homogenous pattern, and 1 in 320 nucleolar pattern, typical of scleroderma.

Other tests showed that she had mycoplasma IgG antibodies, an immune response to a remote infection. The mycoplasma IgM antibody is the response to a recent infection. Often, when patients have a negative mycoplasma antibody titer and are treated with antibiotics that penetrate the cells, those titers become positive; after the antibiotic, dead mycoplasma particles and toxins cause an antigenic stimulus and trigger antibody formation. From the outset, Tylyn's anti-scleroderma 70 antibody was strongly positive. The tests were repeated and verified.

Even though the first titer for mycoplasma IgM, which is

for recent infection, was negative (0 to 1.1 is negative, and above 1.1 is positive), her first titer for lgM was negative at 0.9. The second, on Feb 24, was positive at 1.7, and the third on March 21 was positive at 1.9. The titers were rising in response to the effectiveness of the Minocin. As the lgM antibodies increased progressively, the lgG antibodies, for remote infection, which were positive to begin with at 1.4, started to decrease, to 1.3 on the second drawing and 1.2 by the third in March.

These titers may not appear significantly positive to some, but these two sets of values normally don't go much higher, and Dr. Franco considered them abundant evidence of a mycoplasma infection.

In December, when he ordered a test for mycoplasmas in the circulating white cells (polymerase chain reaction, or PCR, provides a genetic fingerprint of mycoplasma), it was negative. "I have found that the majority of scleroderma patients test negative for mycoplasma PCR in peripheral leukocytes. I don't know if it's because mycoplasmas are so bound to other tissues, including possibly the skin, that they're just not circulating," he says. He compares the white cells to busses; when the mycoplasmas leave the cells, they go to the bus stop, wait for the white cells, board them, and travel to another stop where they get off and penetrate other cells.

The stage may have been set for her scleroderma, Dr. Franco suspected, during Tylyn's pregnancy, perhaps through the suppression of her immune system. However, because she tested positive for mycoplasma pneumonii, there was also a possibility that it began with exposure to that infective agent.

Meanwhile, Tylyn had been in touch with the Scleroderma Foundation, and had agreed to become a spokesperson for building public awareness of her disease. In April, 2000, she was interviewed for a cover story in the Scleroderma Foundation's newsletter. Her picture, showing a flawless face and perfect skin, was a dramatic departure from the image of the disease that readers had come to know and expect.

For Tylyn, however, the problem was not in the picture but the text, a draft of which was sent to her for approval shortly before publication. There was no mention of her therapy, and no indication that she was reversing the normal expectation for her illness by actually getting better. She insisted that if they tell the story at all, they tell it in full, including the treatment, the name of her doctor, even the name and address of The Road Back Foundation. Surprisingly to some, her conditions were met to the letter.

"After four months, she feels dramatically better," the article said of her experience with minocycline. It even raised the possibility that her experience, and similar good results by others, would bring about a reexamination of the role of antibiotics in that disease. It named Dr. Franco, cited the possible role of mycoplasmas, and mentioned the use of minocycline in other connective tissue diseases. "This may be a minority view," the article said, "but unlike the conventional wisdom she had received from other doctors, it gave Tylyn hope."

It gave her more than that. She already felt significantly better, her spirits were improved, and she had recovered most of the energy previously lost to the disease. Although she was on no other medication, the Reynaud's has substantially disappeared and returned in only a minor way during cold spells. All evidence of the sceleroderma in her mouth and face had disappeared, her skin elsewhere had softened dramatically, and the TMJ involvement is steadily returning to normal.

Dr. Franco was unwilling to forecast for any of his patients, but just six months into the therapy he told her he expected that her skin would continue to soften, with a possibility she would be substantially free of the disease within a couple of years.

In June, 2001, Connetics Corp. sponsored a highly visible series of media events as part of Scleroderma
Awareness Month. Hopes ran high for the company's
product Relaxin, then nearing the end of a massive,
nationwide clinical trial. The company's role was trouble-
some to some, however, as the effort seemed designed to
stimulate demand for a product not yet in the marketplace, in advance of an application approval from the FDA
that was expected to issue once the results were unblinded.

This posed a particular dilemma for Tylyn John, whose
role as a Scleroderma Foundation spokesperson required
her to take part in those events while the product was still
unproven. It was all the more problematical because she
had never taken Relaxin or participated in the clinical trial,
and for those reasons she worried that her association with
the event was potentially misleading.

While Tylyn was as hopeful as everyone else that the drug
would prove useful in the treatment of her disease, she
explained over and over that her improvement was not a
result of the sponsor's product. Whenever she had the
chance, she added that she was getting better on minocycline. It was a message not everyone wanted to hear. She was
accompanied on the publicity tour by a doctor who promot-
ed Relaxin extravagantly and at every opportunity, and she
was repeatedly admonished for mentioning the treatment
that had made her well.

The campaign didn't end the way its promoters expected. On October 9th, a Connetics spokesperson announced
in a scleroderma chat on AOL that Relaxin had done no
better in the trials than the placebo. After weeks of intense
media build-up, the failure came as a sad let-down for
those who had bought into the hype.

It was also a shock to participants in the trial. At least one
person in the on-line chat was also a subject in the study, and
now was hearing for the first time that the trial had failed.
The discouraged patient said she had suspected it didn't

work, but she wondered why she hadn't heard the results first from her doctor instead of through this forum on the internet. Then she asked the Connetics researcher if she should unplug the pump by which the Relaxin (or placebo) had been administered. The spokesperson reminded her she had signed a consent form, and that her blood pressure had to be monitored while the drug was slowly withdrawn. Connetics' stock, which had posted a mid-summer high of 28, fell to 4 on news the trials had failed.

A month later, the doctor who accompanied Tylyn on the Relaxin media tour and who repeatedly cautioned her against mentioning the therapy that made her better, was asked about minocycline. Despite his first-hand knowledge of Tylyn's recovery on that therapy, he answered that he never knew of a single patient who had improved on it, and he dismissed minocycline as "quackery."

By the time this edition appears, Tylyn's son Anthony will be five, and Dr. Franco's prophecy has been fulfilled in every particular. Her skin is completely normal. The last of the TMJ and Reynaud's are now behind her. The only remaining evidence of the disease is dental braces, applied to correct a misalignment of her teeth that took place as the result of the tissue damage when her sceleroderma was still raging. With her remission apparently complete, Tylyn stopped taking minocycline in April, 2002. Two months later, she was honored by The Road Back Foundation with the first Vanguard Award for "bringing an awareness of antibiotic therapy to innumerable scleroderma patients through her media presence." Her association with the Scleroderma Foundation ended that same year.

Back in 1998, even before the scleroderma results were presented to the ISRT or published in The Lancet, The Road Back Foundation had begun discussions with Dr. Trentham about the design and scope of an appropriate next step. The first study was vulnerable to criticism on the basis of its size, and a follow-up would be required to gather further data on treatment response in a larger patient population. The announcement of the first results opened the floodgates to an enormous unmet need, and hundreds of patients contacted Dr. Trentham's office for appointments or referrals. Although minocycline still had not received FDA approval in that application, it was ethically appropriate for any doctor who had read the study to prescribe it for scleroderma on the basis of compassionate need. By early 2000, Dr. Trentham and The Road Back directors agreed that his new patient base had attained an appropriate size and composition for such a project.

Unlike the first study, which was physician monitored, the next step was centered on the gathering and statistical analysis of patient information. Enrollment criteria included a diagnosis of any form of scleroderma, not just the systemic or diffuse form that was the focus of the first study; the only exclusions were based on terminal organ involvement. The Foundation's support for this study did not include the cost of medication, which was paid by the subject or an insurer. After an initial appointment in Boston, monitoring of many of the cases took place at long-distance, as Dr. Trentham referred the patient back to a nearer physician. Either way, a detailed questionnaire was used to track disease characteristics in response to treatment. This process was repeated at six-months, one year and two years, with one and two-year follow-up visits in Boston for final physician assessment.

A preliminary report on the results of the first completers of the follow-up—consistent with the positive outcomes in the initial study—was presented at the ISRT meeting in 2002. That report comprises Addendum 2 of this book. Publication of the results from the completed study, following approximately 100 scleroderma patients, is expected in 2004.

*The following is reprinted with permission from* The Lancet *Saturday, November 28, 1998, Volume 352, Number 9142*

## MINOCYCLINE IN NEARLY DIFFUSE SCLERODERMA.

Christine H. Le, Alejandro Morales, David E. Trentham

Based on its efficacy in rheumatoid arthritis[1] and anecdotal evidence, we did an open trial of minocycline in early diffuse scleroderma. Patients satisfied criteria for the diagnosis of scleroderma[2] and did not have additional rheumatic disease. Inclusion criteria were clinical systemic sclerosis on the extremities proximal to the elbow and knee and on the trunk below the clavicles, and disease duration of 3 years or less from the onset of the first symptoms, including Raynaud's phenomenon, as determined by the patient's rheumatologist. Exclusion criteria included internal-organ damage.

Patients were evaluated at 3-month intervals for 1 year. Medications for Raynaud's and gastrointestinal-tract disturbances were continued. Patients on treatments that might modify scleroderma had a 1-month washout period. Minocycline was started at 50 mg twice daily, taken with water on an empty sctomach; the dose was increased to 100 mg twice daily after 1 month. At each visit, a previously validated total skin score (TSS) was determined by palpation of the skin at 17 surface areas and was graded: 0=normal, 1-thickened skin, 2=thickened, unable to move, and 3=thickened, unable to pinch; maximum possible TSS was 51.[3] Response in TSS was defined as a more than 35% decrease at 12 months. To measure overall well being, a patient and physician 10 cm visual analogue scale (VAS) was used: 0 cm=could not be better, 10 cm=could not be worse.[4] Response in VAS was arbitrarily defined as more than 35% decreased at 12 months.

Eleven patients, all diagnosed by at least one independent rheumatologist, were enrolled. Patients number 1, 4, and 11 washed off penicillamine and 2, methotrexate (table). A single observer (CHL) did the evaluations except for the final two visits of patient 11. At the end of 1 year, four patients had complete resolution of their skin disease and their final TSS was 0 (table). In three of these four patients, patient and physician VAS scores improved to 0. In two of the 11 patients, there was no improvement in TSS. In one of these two patients, there was a significant improvement in VAS scores.

Five patients did not complete the study; two with renal crisis, one died of adenocarcinoma, and two were non-compliant. Adverse reactions included oral yeast infection in one patient and two episodes of vaginal yeast infection in another. One patient developed nausea and dizziness for the first two weeks. On initial testing, serum concentrations of the adhesion molecules, ICAM-1, VCAM-1, and E-selectin[5] were elevated in patients 11, 10, and 9. Changes did not occur during the trial.

No accepted reversal treatment for scleroderma exists. Although the mechanism of action is unknown, minocycline should undergo larger-scale study in scleroderma.

*Supported in part by a grant from The Road Back Foundation and NIH Grant M01-RR01032, Beth Israel Deaconess Medical Center, East Campus General Clinical Research Center. Miocycline was supplied by Wyeth-Ayerst Laboratories.*

1. Tilley BC, Alarcón GS, Heyse SP, et al. Minocycline in rheumatoid arthritis: a 48-week, double-blind, placebo-controlled trial. *Ann Intern Med* 1995; **122:** 81–89.
2. Subcommittee for Scleroderma Criteria of the American Rheumatism Association Diagnostic and Therapeutic Criteria Committee. Preliminary criteria for the classification of systemic sclerosis (scleroderma). *Arthritis Rheum* 1980; **30:** 581–90.
3. Brennan P, Silman A, Black C, et al. Reliability of skin

involvement measures in scleroderma. *Br J Rheymatol* 1992; **31:** 457–60

4. Van Den Hoogen FHJ, Boerbooms AMT, Swaak AJG, Rasker JJ, van Lier HJJ, Van De Putte LBA. Comparison of methotrexate with placebo in the treatment of systemic sclerosis: a 24 week randomized double-blind trial followed by a 24 week observational trial. *Br J Rheymatol* 1996; **35:** 364–72

5. Gruschwitz MS, Hornstein OP, Van den Driesch P. Correlation of soluble adhesion molecules in the peripheral blood of scleroderma patients with their in situ expression and with disease activity. *Arthritis Rheum* 1995; **38:** 184–89

**Beth Israel Deaconess Medical Center and Harvard Medical School, 330 Brookline Avenue, Boston, MA 02215, USA** (DE Trentham; e-mail drentha@bidmc.harvard.edu)

| Patient | Time | | | | | Outcome/adverse events |
|---|---|---|---|---|---|---|
| | Baseline | 3* | 6 | 9 | 12 | |
| 1 | 43/8·2/9·8† | 26/1·8/8·4 | 40/2·4/9·2 | 34/8·6/7·7 | 40/8·5/8·8 | Vaginal yeast |
| 2 | 33/2·8/4 | 22/4·8/3·7 | 20/0·3/05 | 4/0/0 | 0/0/0 | Completed |
| 3 | 43/5/5·5 | - | - | - | - | Renal crisis at 2 months |
| 4 | 15/2/1·8 | 7/5/5·2 | 0/2/0·8 | 0/0/0 | 0/0/0 | Completed |
| 5 | 32/2·8/5·5 | 17/0/4·8 | 10/2·1/2/2·2 | - | - | Died at 7 m |
| 6 | 20/7·8/7 | 15/2·8/4 | 13/2·5/2·5 | 10/2·4/2·5 | - | Did not return |
| 7 | 25/4·7/3·2 | 5/0·3/0·5 | 5/0·7/0·2 | 0/0/0 | 0/0/0 | Completed |
| 8 | 32/4·8/7·4 | _ | - | - | - | Renal crisis at 2 m |
| 9 | 20/0·9/0·9 | 4/6·9/6·6 | 1/4·4/3·8 | 0/0·9/0·9 | 0/0·9/0·3 | Oral yeast |
| 10 | 33/5·7/8·2 | 35/7·8/7·8 | - | - | - | Changed to IV minocycline‡ |
| 11 | 15/2·5/2·2 | 11/3/1·5 | 9/2·0/1·9 | 13/2·9/1·2 | 11/1·4/1 | Completed |

*Months into treatment
†Total skin score/patient global score/physician global score
‡Patient decision and performed elsewhere

# ADDENDUM 2:

# The ISRT Preview of Long-Term Effects

---

*The following is an abstract presented at the 8th Biennial Congress of the International Society for Rheumatic Therapies in Washington, DC, in April, 2002. Peer-reviewed publication of the complete survey is expected in 2004.*

## SERIAL SURVEY OF THE LONG-TERM EFFECT OF MINOCYCLINE ON SCLERODERMA.

**David E. Trentham, M.D. and Roselynn Dynesius-Trentham, M.S.**

Since 1999 we have attempted to follow longitudinally, in a rolling format of enrollment, more than 177 patients with the diagnosis of scleroderma—diffuse, limited or morphea—who either have been seen in our clinic or have been referred by their physicians to participate in the study. This study is a serial survey seeking to assess disease characteristics, progression of disease and the long-term effects of minocycline (Minocin) on their disorder and their approximately 6 month intervals. This report describes briefly the outcome of the 27 patients that have achieved more than a year of follow-up and have been compliant with reporting.

Sixteen and 10 patients have diffuse and limited forms, respectively, of scleroderma and 1 had a

PSS/overlap syndrome. Three of the 27 have never been on Minocin (disease very mild—1) or for only a short time because of toxicity issues (severe nausea—1, hepatic cholestatic jaundice—1) but have decided to participate for a balanced view of disease progression. By patient report benefit to oral Minocin 100 mg bid on an empty stomach was graded as "too early," none, a little, moderate amount, or a lot.

In the 1st survey, 15 patients concluded that Minocin was helping a lot, 7 thought that it was helping a moderate amount, 3 judged no benefit, and 2 stated that it was too early to know.

In the 2nd survey, responses in these categories were 21 (a lot), 2 (moderate amount), 1 (between little and moderate amount) and 3 for no benefit.

In the 3rd questionnaire the results are 21 (a lot), 3 (moderate) and 3 (none).

Response to Minocin was also graded by patient global assessment, based on a visual analog scale ranging from 0 (very well) to 10 (very poor). Mean scores were 3.44, 2.44, and 2.01 for the 3 surveys.

The majority of 1st questionnaires were derived from patients who had been on Minocin for an extended period (mean=11.23 months at baseline) so that their responses were not representative of a pre-treatment state and increased benefit over time was more modest than expected. Side effects to Minocin were those already recognized and described for the compound. The most commonly associated problems were dizziness and nausea.

In summary the majority of patients reporting indicated that minocycline is, in general, well tolerated and is capable of helping some patients with diffuse and limited scleroderma.

# INDEX

## *HOW TO HELP*

---

The scleroderma studies described in this book were performed at Beth Israel Deaconess Hospital, a teaching hospital at Harvard Medical School, under the sponsorship of The Road Back Foundation.

The Foundation was established as a not-for-profit 501(c)3 corporation in 1993. Staffed mainly by volunteers, it supports studies and clinical trials of antibiotics in connective tissue disease, and also provides the latest comprehensive information on this therapy free of charge to patients and doctors around the world.

To help support ongoing and future research into scleroderma and other connective tissue diseases with your tax-deductible contributions, or to obtain current information on antibiotic research and treatment, write to:

The Road Back Foundation
Box 447
Orleans, MA 02653

Voice mail calls at (614) 224-1556 will be returned. Visit the Foundation's web site at www.roadback.org.

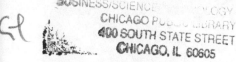
BUSINESS/SCIENCE/TECHNOLOGY DIVISION
CHICAGO PUBLIC LIBRARY
400 SOUTH STATE STREET
CHICAGO, IL 60605

R02018 86613

**to** Thomas McPherson Brown, M.D.,
Pat Ganger,
**and** David Trentham, M.D.